HEALTH TO VITALITY

HEALTH TO VITALITY

Liberate Yourself From the Shackles of
Traditional Health Care & Empower Yourself to
Create a Life of Vitality & Fulfillment

Matthew LaBosco

For more information, email matt@healthtovitality.com

ISBN: 979-8-88759-072-1 (paperback)
ISBN: 979-8-88759-073-8 (ebook)

Vitality[1]

- *Exuberant physical strength or mental vigor*
- *The capacity for continuation of a meaningful*
- *and purposeful existence*
- *The power to live and grow*

Health[2]

- *The state of being free from illness or injury*

Stop struggling to be healthy
Learn how to create Vitality

[1]   The Free Dictionary (2022)
[2]   Google – Dictionary Box (2022)

BONUS #1

You will find that this book contains a ton of information, strategies, techniques, and tools that will be VERY different from what you have read in any other book. To help you assimilate and apply the information, I have created a series of videos that you can use as a way to supplement and support you on this journey.

All you need to do is go to:

HEALTHTOVITALITY.COM/VIDEOS

It is absolutely free. Enjoy

Health to Vitality
Summary Videos

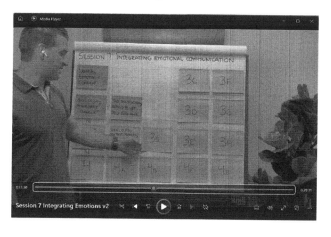

Dedications

Without question, the first people I want to thank and dedicate this book to are my parents. I'm not sure what I did in my past lives to be rewarded with these incredible human beings, but it must have been something. The unconditional love, encouragement, dedication, and support they have provided me my entire life is beyond comprehension. Without their relentless love and support, there is no way I would have been able to create this book and my incredible life. Thank you, Mom and Dad.

And to my mentors, teachers, and colleagues, I cherish the time I have spent with every one of you. Everyone listed below has played a significant and, in some cases, a critical role in my journey by offering their love, care, guidance, support, and knowledge to me. I would not be the man I am today without each of you making these priceless contributions. For that, I am eternally grateful.

Lenny Parracino, Harvey Green, Dana Roberts, Josh Guerrero, Dr. Yoshi Rahm, Dodie Anderson, and Dr. Ray Peat

A Special Thank You

To my incredible wife, Eve. So much of what I have written in this book we have discovered, grown, and persevered through together. I cannot express the amount of appreciation and gratitude I have in my heart for having you in my life as a partner, friend, consultant, teacher, wife, and mother of my children. I am truly blessed to have you by my side. Love you.

Contents

Note to Reader

This book is for individuals who are frustrated and unwilling to settle for the limitations that our healthcare system and the health paradigm provide. And it is definitely for people who have been told nothing more can be done for their situation besides more medication, surgeries, or coping strategies. I believe the information in this book would bankrupt our current medical, health, and wellness models if applied by everyone. The principles I share in this book are the things big pharma and the medical system do *not* want you to know or practice.

I grew up in the medical model—my dad is a physician, and my mom is a nurse practitioner. Like many health professionals, my parents dedicated their lives to helping and serving their patients. They can fulfill this because of their enormous hearts, compassion, and love despite being handicapped by the system. The unfortunate reality is that the systems and institutions they work in are neither conducive to nor aligned with creating *vitality* for the public. The system is designed to keep you "free from injury or illness." My dad once told me he had about eight minutes to figure out why someone had a headache because that was the time the system allotted. That put things into perspective for me by making it clear that the system was set up to treat the symptoms and move people through the process. Unfortunately, there is not a lot of money in keeping people healthy. Most of the financial benefits are tied to curing diseases and fixing things that are broken. The most money is made not by curing illness and disease but by creating treatments for an illness that the patient will need for the rest of their life.

When my wife, Eve, and I were preparing for the birth of our first child, I had an eye-opening experience. We attended a pre-birth workshop at the University of Southern California Verdugo Hills Hospital. I'll never forget walking into that room with twenty pregnant women and seeing the snacks and beverages laid out for everyone. The table was filled with bags of chips, processed deli meats, and sodas. Processed foods? For pregnant women?!

I was so shocked that I could barely focus on what they were saying and recommending. How could I possibly listen to the advice of these individuals when they were serving processed food to pregnant women? Researchers have found that processed foods contain certain preservatives that change nervous system development in the fetal brain, creating a higher risk of autism.[3] Had we been trapped by an institution that was supposed to keep us healthy but didn't know how? Then I remembered how the traditional system defined health—the absence of disease. It was moments like this, I realized that educating myself and taking health into my own hands would be necessary. I needed to create a new paradigm, one that was anchored to a different set of principles and guidelines. And so, my journey of birthing the Vitality Principles began.

Before the age of twenty-two I had five orthopedic injuries requiring surgery. Throughout my life I have suffered from depression, overwhelm, anxiety, and periods of feeling purposeless. Eve and I have both struggled with different inflammatory, systemic, and autoimmune ailments throughout the years. The only solutions the medical models ever offered us were medications, surgeries, and ways to cope, settle, or numb ourselves through the pain. What was offered

---

[3]   Brookes Megan (2019)

didn't even help us to create good health, let alone open us up to living lives sparkling with vitality.

In this book, I will share and review vitality principles in the context of movement, the systemic system, and mindset. My goal is to provide you with a solid paradigm that offers to

1. Empower you with the resources to create the most fulfilling and meaningful life possible and eliminate the idea that there is something wrong with you

2. Give you the ability to trust yourself and provide a way to use the educational and healthcare system instead of being enslaved by it

3. Provide you with a framework that you can use to get started on your exploration of these principles so that *you can use them* to create what you choose

This book is the distillation of the knowledge gained during the twenty-year journey that Eve and I have been on as we have navigated through our struggles with the physical, systemic, and mental aspects of health and wellness. It also comes from our experiences supporting thousands of individuals at our Vitality Center in Southern California, our private practices, and the students in our online courses. Our mission is to create a *new* system, framework, and network of like-minded professionals that provide people with a foundation they can use to build the most meaningful and fulfilling life possible. I am honored and grateful to be included in your life's journey and excited to support you on that journey from *Health to Vitality*.

Yours in Vitality,
Matthew LaBosco

THE DAY
EVERYTHING
CHANGED

Chapter 1

"X-RAYS LOOK GOOD"

Let me give you a little more context about my background and me. I was number four of five kids born to a medical physician and nurse practitioner in central New Jersey. It is safe to say I grew up in the medical model framework and I am very grateful for the perks that it provided me. My parents were very loving and did everything in their power to keep us happy, healthy, and strong.

I was a three-sport athlete and spent most of my time playing sports. There was not a day during my childhood when I was not in the middle of some sports season. Baseball, soccer, and basketball were my primary sports, and I loved playing them all.

Being this active meant managing all the aches, pains, and injuries that come with being a three sport athlete. It started with baseball. I played Little League for as long as I could. I started when I was old enough to hold a bat, all the way up until high school. Strangely enough, my Little League baseball team was the Red Sox, even though I was born and raised a diehard Yankee fan. You can imagine my inner turmoil. Anyway, there was a four to five year stretch during my Little League career where a teammate of mine and I pitched every other game and never lost. And when we were not pitching, we were playing shortstop. Needless to say, our arms didn't have too many days off. Did we have some soreness? Were we icing our arms down a little more each season? Sure, but it wasn't stopping us, and we loved it!

Well, all good things must come to an end, and they sure did. Fast-forward to high school, time for baseball tryouts. I was excited to show my friends and the coach that they had a ball player on their hands. A buddy of mine and I grabbed our mitts and started playing catch to warm up. As I took my first few throws, I felt a twinge in my elbow. Weird, I thought, but whatever. I was sure it was nothing. As we continued throwing, I noticed that the way I was throwing the baseball was changing. I was throwing the ball without bending my elbow. I continued throwing, hoping I just needed to warm up, but it only got worse. It got to the point where I couldn't find a way to throw the ball and effectively get it over to my teammate. This was the beginning of my elbow problems. Over the next few years, I was diagnosed with golfer's elbow and tennis elbow. You can imagine how confusing that was to me. It turns out that golfer's and tennis elbow diagnoses were just references to the location of the injury. When the injury is on the outside of the elbow, it is called tennis elbow. When the injury is on the inside of the elbow, it is called golfer's elbow. My elbow hurt all over.

Eventually, playing baseball became too painful, but thankfully I was able to continue playing basketball and soccer. I made the varsity soccer team as a freshman and made varsity basketball as a sophomore in high school. I also started weight training in junior high because that was what I was told would enable me to avoid more injuries and improve my overall performance. Furthermore, I was also secretly holding out some hope to return to the baseball field. I was told I needed to build more core and upper body strength, and so I did. I hit the gym religiously for the next six years.

During this time, the elbow continued to get worse. I started doing physical therapy and taking some over the counter antiinflammatory medications, but it got to the point that nothing was helping anymore. It was bad enough that it eventually impacted my ability to shoot a basketball. My sophomore year in highschool, I got my first surgery on my right elbow.

It was an "easy" surgery. Fortunately, they were able to do what was needed with an arthroscopic procedure. This meant they didn't have to create a large incision and were able to get in there with a few small puncture openings leading to a faster recovery.

After the surgery and rehabilitation of my elbow, I was ready to return to playing soccer and basketball. Baseball was no longer an option despite all the rehab and surgery—I was told never to throw a ball again. I was super bummed but was also grateful that I was able to shoot a basketball and didn't need my elbow to play soccer.

I wish I could tell you it was smooth sailing from there, but it wasn't. My entire high school career was plagued with knee problems and chronic ankle sprains. I was in and out of the high school trainer's office every day, doing rehab on my ankles, getting my ankles taped up, and then slapping on ankle braces. I was there five days a week, strengthening all the muscles around my ankle to create more stability in that region. I sprained my ankles so much that by the time I was in college, I was told I needed total reconstruction on my left ankle.

I managed to tape and limp myself through high school basketball and nearly finished my senior year. Unfortunately, I sprained my ankle very badly and was unable to complete the last month of the season and finished about forty points away from scoring 1000 points in my high school career. It would be an understatement to say it was a frustrating end to my athletic career. I did, however, get recruited to play basketball by a division III school called Tufts University, but I never saw the court for a game because I was always injured. I eventually transferred from Tufts and graduated from Rutgers College in New Jersey.

At this point, my interests in the body, specifically orthopedics, training, rehabilitation, and fitness, were amplified. I interned with an orthopedic surgeon for an entire summer, watching and observing all kinds of orthopedic assessments and surgeries. I also took every strength and conditioning, physical rehabilitation, personal training course, webinar, and class I could find.

I was determined to strengthen my body so I wouldn't be so injury-prone. I worked out religiously and gave it 100 percent each day. I spent tens of thousands of dollars attending seminars with top sports performance experts, learning everything I could about strength and conditioning and Olympic weightlifting. I was a common fixture at the seminars of performance coach gurus like Charles Poloquin, Ian King, and Paul Chek. I became certified as an Olympic Weightlifting Coach with USA Weightlifting, a Certified Strength and Conditioning Specialist with the National Strength and Conditioning Association, and a Performance Enhancement Specialist and Corrective Exercise Specialist with the National Academy of Sports Medicine. I applied all this knowledge and achieved a level of performance I had never reached before. I weighed about 210 pounds and was about 8 percent body fat. I was the strongest I had ever been, bench pressing 385 pounds and squatting 450 pounds.

As far as my elbow was concerned, I still had discomfort here and there but managed the pain by doing my physical therapy exercises and taking the occasional anti-inflammatory medication. Good old Advil was one of my staples, but my absolute favorite medication was an anti-inflammatory called Vioxx. I used to refer to it as a miracle drug. Anytime my elbow was hurting, I'd pop one of those pills, and *viola*! I was healed! I'd load up more weight and bang out a few more sets. I was even able to throw a baseball again! Then I was told that I shouldn't take too much of this particular medication because it seemed to have major side effects. Eventually, it was pulled off the market after a 2004 study that showed Vioxx caused an increased risk of serious cardiovascular events, such as stroke and heart attack.[4]

Around this time, I had a life-changing experience at the Sports Club LA on the Upper East Side in New York City.

It was a normal Tuesday morning, and I was getting ready for my workout before working with clients as a personal trainer. I was going for a PR (personal record) on the military press that day. The military press is an exercise where you sit on a bench with a backrest and press a barbell overhead. I was about to lift the most weight I had ever attempted to press over my head from a seated position, and I was feeling good! As I prepared to lift the 315 pounds, I inhaled deeply. My friend helped me unrack the weight and spotted me as I guided the bar down to my upper chest. As I slowly exhaled, I began straightening my arms, pressing the weight toward the sky. With my friend's hands spotting me and his encouraging words, I was able to lock my elbows and extend that 315 pounds over my head. I then guided the barbell back to the rack, stood up, and felt like I had arrived. Man, it felt good to press that much weight over my head, especially after all the injuries I had sustained through playing baseball, basketball, and soccer. Maybe there was hope for me. Maybe I wasn't as broken as I thought I was.

---

[4] NPR (2005–2007)

And then, it happened.

I took a few steps away from the upright bench, and my entire right arm seized. I couldn't move it—it felt like my lower arm was dangling from my elbow. It was excruciating to let my arm hang there—I needed to support it with my other hand to tolerate the pain. The only thing that went through my head at that moment was, "I destroyed my elbow."

Convinced that my elbow had exploded and I needed surgery ASAP, I called my orthopedic surgeon (who, at this point, was on my speed dial) to find out when we could do the necessary second surgery on this elbow to fix it.

I got in to see him that next week. After listening to what happened, evaluating my X-rays, and performing his orthopedic assessment, he was ready to tell me what was wrong and how we would fix it. The words that came out of his mouth in that moment, are words I will never forget. They completely changed the trajectory of my life.

"I don't see anything wrong with your elbow. X-rays look good."

"What?!" I said, in complete shock. "How could that possibly be? I can barely move this thing, and it even hurts when it's not moving!"

His only suggestion was to "go in there" and see if he could find anything.

I was dumbfounded. It just didn't make any sense. How could he possibly tell me there was nothing wrong with my elbow? It was pretty clear that there was something seriously wrong.

And then it hit me—doctors don't have all the answers. Not only did they not have all the answers, but it was quite unfair for me to expect they would and to demand that they give me an answer immediately.

I thanked him and told him I was going to think about it but that I would hold off on the surgery for now.

As I left the orthopedics' office that day, I realized that the current model of physical rehabilitation, orthopedics, and fitness might not be able to help me. It seemed like the paradigm they were operating under had huge limitations. I had many unanswered questions and wasn't sure where to go to get the answers, but I was determined to find them.

This day marked the beginning of my quest to find a new way.

In the next chapter, I will break down the limitations of the health paradigm. Specifically, I will reveal the foundational principles of the healthcare model in three spaces: 1-physical rehabilitation and fitness, 2- systemic care and nutrition, and 3- mindset and stress. I will take you through the journey that Eve and I have taken down these three spaces and share the flaws in the traditional model that left us with no other options but medication, surgeries, and coping strategies.

In the chapters that follow (chapters 3-7), I will introduce a new framework that I've developed and anchored to a vitality paradigm. A paradigm that doesn't require coping strategies, numbing pain, or treating symptoms. Instead, this new paradigm that is anchored to principles that focus on the big picture, leveraging the body's innate power to heal and addressing root causes. A framework that has you partner with your body's incredible ability to live a life of meaning, purpose, and fulfillment - a life of vitality.

My wife, Eve, and I have applied the principles in this book for over twenty years and feel better today than we did in our twenties. I have no limitations to what I can do today, including throwing a baseball.

LIMITATIONS TO PURSUING "HEALTHY"

Chapter 2

"Houston ... We Have A Problem"

*Part I: The Problems with the Healthcare
Paradigm For Physical Rehabilitation & Fitness*

So, I'm Not a Walking Cadaver?

The experience I had that day in the office of my orthopedic surgeon ignited a passion and determination to get to the bottom of what was going on with my body. I knew my questions were not going to be easy to answer and that I was going to have to figure it out by piecing things together myself. It became abundantly clear through my experience that there were some major holes in the way that people were rehabilitated and treated for orthopedic injuries. I was ready to embark on the journey and coincidentally, early on in this journey, I met someone who was on a similar mission.

I met my wife Eve at a local gym when I was in my senior year of college. We were both trainers, and we both had the same passion for learning about health, wellness, and fitness. We were also passionate about sharing that with others. We always enjoyed each other's company and started becoming good friends. Believe it or not, our relationship grew to the next level thanks to one of my ankle injuries. I was playing basketball, by myself, on the court in the gym where we both worked. I was shooting around and when I went to jump, in an attempt to dunk the basketball, I completely rolled my ankle again. I sprained it so badly that I could not walk—it was one of my worst ankle sprains ever. Eve, who was working then, came in and found me lying on the court, unable to stand. All part of my plan to get more of her attention, of course - ok, not really. She quickly helped me to my feet and took me to the emergency room. She spent the entire eight hours with me at the hospital and continued caring for me while I got back on my feet over the following few weeks. We spent a lot of time with each other, and it was clear there was something special about her and our connection. We ended up getting married two years later, in August of 2002.

We both continued our journeys with health and fitness. Eve worked in the spa industry as a manager and massage therapist. She also continued to do some personal training and nutritional consulting on the side. I continued educating myself in every way I could. In addition to all the courses I took on physical rehabilitation, fitness, anatomy, physiology, and orthopedic injuries, I also sought out clinicians who were getting results with individuals whom no one else could help. I latched on to them as much as they would let me. At one point, Eve and I moved across the country so I could apprentice and learn from one of my most influential mentors, a clinician by the name of Lenny Parracino. Lenny is currently one of the most sought-after rehabilitation specialists in California—so much so that the NBA's Los Angeles Clippers basketball team has hired him to take care of their million dollar athletes.

After learning from brilliant clinicians like Lenny, it became abundantly clear why the traditional model of physical rehabilitation, like orthopedics, chiropractic, and physical therapy, had the limitations I was seeing. The biggest limitation to these approaches is the way they were taught human anatomy. All the anatomy taught in traditional medical models is based on studying a human cadaver, otherwise known as cadaveric anatomy.

So, what is the problem with this, you ask? Well, a cadaver is obviously not alive and not moving. We are observing a system that is completely turned off and attempting to evaluate how it works when it is "turned on." We dissect the parts of this system and then make assumptions about how they integrate as a whole. The great philosopher Aristotle pointed out the major limitations to this approach thousands of years ago with his famous quote, "the whole is greater than the sum of its parts."[5]

When you pick up the latest muscle anatomy book or simply google any muscle, it will tell you the origin and insertion of the muscle and then tell you its function. Take the hamstrings as an example. If you look up the function of the hamstrings, it will tell you that it primarily flexes the knee. Because of this, every gym on the planet has a leg curl machine that has a picture of a hamstring on it to indicate that you are working that muscle.

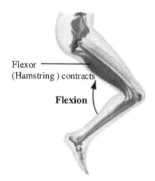

Flexor
(Hamstring) contracts

Flexion

Fig 1 Hamstring Muscle flexing the knee joint [6]

---

[5]   Aristotle cited by Upton Joseph et al. (2014)
[6]   Benazzouz Ahlem et al. (2019)

To say that the primary role of the hamstring is to flex the knee is an insult to the hamstring. This would be the equivalent of saying the primary function of a mom is to change diapers! Are you kidding me? Sure, the hamstring *can* flex the knee, just like mom *can* change a diaper, but not only is it something it does at times, it does an infinite number of much more dynamic and essential things. Thinking that this is the primary function of the hamstring and strengthening it in this way, means we don't understand the hamstring at all.

What is the function of the hamstring, then? Just like the function of every other muscle in the body, the answer is "it depends." It depends on many variables, including the context, the position of the body, and the tasks being performed. It is way more intricate and complicated than "it flexes the knee." In certain movements, the hamstring is actually extending the knee, like in walking. Therefore if you have a hamstring strain that hurts when walking, jogging, or running, the only way to properly rehabilitate it would be to understand what the hamstrings are doing when you walk, jog, or run.

This is the main flaw of the traditional physical therapy and fitness model. Their entire approach is based on the anatomy of a dead person. Consider the most popular core exercise—the crunch (Fig 2a). The crunch exercise was based on the fact that the rectus abdominis (Fig 2b) (the six-pack muscle) originates from the xiphoid process and inserts into the pubic synthesis.

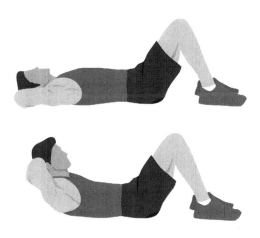

Fig 2a. Crunch Exercise

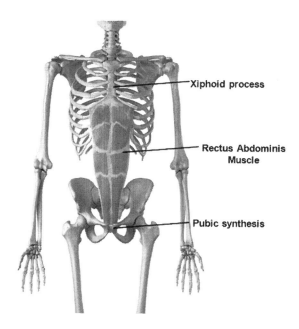

Fig 2b. Rectus Abdominis Muscle

Based on its origin and insertion, it is then deduced that the function of this muscle is to flex the trunk. What I find fascinating about this advice is that this exercise trains the body to get into the same position we are all trying to avoid—rounded shoulders and forward head, known more commonly as "poor posture." The interesting thing about the rectus abdominis is that the majority of its action happens when the trunk is in extension, not flexion, like a volleyball player spiking a volleyball (Fig 2c).

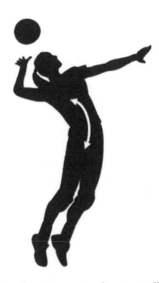

Fig 2c. Rectus Abdominis extending in Volleyball Spike

I could go through every muscle in the body and show you the similar examples. As a matter of fact, all you need to do is go to your local gym, and you will see a circuit set up for people to give them a "full body workout," which will consist of approximately 10–15 machines that isolate 10–15 different muscles. The problem is that the only time the body performs these types of movements is when it is locked into a position on a machine, forcing them to work in unnatural, isolated positions doing unnatural, isolated movements. These types of isolated exercises are the biggest reasons I have been busy rehabbing people for the last twenty years.

The best analogy I have to show you the dysfunction of this approach is an orchestra. Imagine you were the conductor of an orchestra and you learned the best way to train your musicians was the same way we have been taught to train our muscles. You would need to take every musician in the orchestra, isolate them in separate rooms, and get them to play as loudly as they can. After each and every instrument has been isolated to play as loudly as possible to the complete exhaustion of the musicians, you then bring them back into one room and ask them to play music together. Imagine what the result of that would be - a lot of noise. This is what we have when we do this to the body—the "noise" for the body is an injury. The approach to isolate muscles and get them to scream as loudly as possible was very effective at getting a muscle to grow and become leaner, but not at creating fluid, efficient movement patterns.

One other important piece to note. When you are actually looking at the musculature of a cadaver, it looks *nothing* like the muscle charts in the anatomy books. When doing cadaveric dissection, you must work really hard to isolate each muscle and identify its origin and insertion. It is even more complicated trying to figure out how each muscle works in isolation from the other muscles and soft tissues. This should be the first BIG clue as to why this has serious implications. The body would never choose to isolate one muscle and ask it to do all the work.

These were the ways Eve and I were taught to train ourselves and our clients. It was starting to make more and more sense why we, and our clients, had the aches and pains we had.

Part II: The Problems with the Healthcare Paradigm for Nutrition & Systemic Care

Fill it up ... Zero Octane Gas Please

Through my time learning, exploring, and applying the movement principles I will be sharing with you in the next chapter, I was able to successfully rehabilitate my elbow without any surgery or medication. I was back to working out, playing pick-up basketball and softball 2–4 days a week, and functioning with no more pain. As I felt like I was getting a better handle on my physical ailments, my focus shifted to optimizing and learning more about nutrition and managing my systemic state. During our early years together, Eve and I struggled with some of the normal systemic things, like sustaining energy levels throughout the day, occasional headaches, and getting sick a little more than we would have liked. Similar to movement, I took a deep dive into studying the latest approaches and philosophies of nutrition. As you may have noticed yourself when it comes to nutrition, there are a lot of people telling us to do a lot of different things. For every person who tells you blueberries prevent cancer, you can find 2–3 people who will tell you that blueberries cause cancer. It is super confusing and when things are confusing, I put my focus on getting to the foundation or principles of the recommendations being made.

The most common paradigm in the world of nutrition is what I call the "diet and exercise" model. The fundamental principle of the diet and exercise model is the manipulation of caloric input and output. Essentially, you consume fewer calories than you burn to accomplish the objective of losing weight. The problem I started to notice was this model started trickling into the idea of health.

Because so many people were overweight, the diet and exercise model became the healthy option. So, every recommendation that was created and deemed "healthy" was aligned with this paradigm. This is why you see a picture of a salad on the cover of almost every health magazine. Salads are extremely low in caloric value which somehow has made them "healthy."

Let's pause for a moment and define what a calorie is. A calorie is a unit of energy. These units of energy are what food is supposed to deliver to the system for it to function optimally. I like to think of the number of calories in my food as being similar to the amount of octane in gasoline. Would you put zero octane fuel in your car? (Fig 3) Would you put water in your gas tank so that it is full? I think it is safe to say you would not. The difference between you and your car is your body will still run on zero calories to a point, but your car will not run without fuel. If your car worked like your body and it ran out of fuel, it would start using itself as fuel. It would turn the body parts of your car into fuel, and eventually, the car would fall apart on the road piece by piece. This is what happens to the body when we deprive it of the necessary calories. It can be a serious problem when not addressed. The process of breaking down the body for fuel is called catabolism. *Catabolism* is "the breakdown of complex molecules in living organisms to form simpler ones, together with the release of energy, and is also associated with destructive metabolism."[7] When we are put in this catabolic state through a lack of calories, the body starts to break down its lean tissue, like muscle, which can lead to a variety of problems over time.

---

[7]   Oxford Languages (2022)

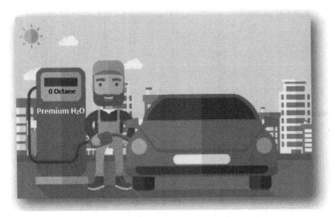

Fig 3: Man Filling Up Car with Water

Now, don't get me wrong, there are definitely plenty of circumstances where someone is eating too many calories, and quantity needs to be addressed. What I have found, however, is a correlation between overeating and consuming high volumes of "empty calories." Empty calories are foods that are very low in nutritional value and keep you wanting more. Now typically "empty calories" refer to processed foods with fake sugar, fat, and salt that trick the body into feeling it received some essential resources like glucose, sodium, and fatty acids. Foods that contain artificial sweeteners like corn syrups, and fake fats like carrageenan, are an example of these types of foods. Not only have these additives been linked to many unwanted side effects[8], but they will also lead to overeating because the body is left still needing the resources it needs. There are some "healthy" foods that I put into the empty calorie category as well—food like salads, other green leafy foods, and vegetables. Because there are zero to very few calories in these types of foods, eating them leaves you "full" but still hungry and with intense cravings for sweet and salty

---

[8]   Peat Ray (1995)

foods. When you start eating high-quality caloric foods that have *real* sugar, salt, and fat in them, the need for volume often disappears.

Now, although the diet and exercise model was a significant influence on determining which foods were healthy, there was also another primary influence that guided healthy eating. This was the government's recommendations made through the USDA. Now from a government's perspective, I can understand why the recommendations were made. I would imagine that the goal of the government was to make sure everyone was fed. The name of the game was quantity, not quality. The USDA Food Pyramid[9] recommends that over 40 percent of our caloric intake come from bread, cereal, rice, and pasta. Essentially, eat grains. Grains are the cheapest and easiest way to feed the most people. Grains provide 80 percent of the world's caloric needs.[10] When you factor in the government's recommendation to eat 40 percent grains, it isn't a shock that people are overweight, and therefore the diet and exercise model was created. I hope you can see by now that neither one of these frameworks would ever produce vitality. The Food Pyramid is all about quantity, not quality and the diet and exercise model is about deprivation. It creates a vicious never-ending cycle. (Fig 4)

[9] Wikipedia. "Food Pyramid." (2022)
[10] Amadeo Kimberly (2022)

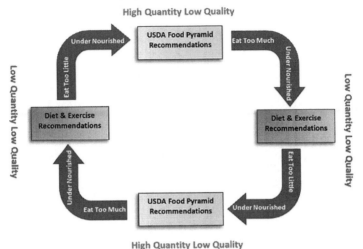

Fig 4: Vicious Cycle of Diet & Exercise and USDA Food Recommendations

Not only is vitality not possible with this model, but eating this way creates an infinite number of side effects. Every systemic disease that you can think of can be correlated to a poor diet, whether by directly causing it or by exacerbating conditions. The side effects on hormones, metabolism, digestion, energy levels, sleep, sex drive, recovery, and our immune system are in the hundreds of thousands and counting. One example I know many people can relate to is what eliminating grains from your diet can do for health problems. There are numerous symptoms I as well as many other people I've worked with have eliminated by simply eliminating grains. Symptoms like stomach pain, gas, diarrhea, constipation, periods of fatigue, brain fog, and headaches. The one symptom that was the most eye-opening to me was the elimination of joint pain throughout my body. I frequently experienced achy non-specific joint pain and discomfort, none of which was correlated to any specific type of movement. Once I eliminated grains from my diet and implemented the vitality principles for eating, the joint pain disappeared. To this day, if I eat too many grains, I can start to feel the inflammation in my body increase, and my joints will be the first to let me know I've overdone it.

The USDA Food Pyramid, just like the diet and exercise model, doesn't provide us with resources to know vitality, or even health. However, it does make us very sick. (Fig 5) It also conveniently provides a market for thousands of businesses to address all the side effects of eating this way. Businesses that offer you gluten-free products are some of the biggest. According to alliedmarketresearch.com, the gluten-free product markets are estimated to hit 7.5 billion dollars by 2027![11] But there are plenty of other companies and industries that have emerged—essentially, any company promising you more energy, better sleep, higher sex drive, relief from digestive disorders, and so on. This entire approach would be analogous to poisoning a tree slowly so it was able to survive, but its leaves, branches, bark, and every other component of the tree needed constant attention and care. And instead of not poisoning the tree, we created an industry that specialized in treating all the different ailments that the poison creates—a leaf doctor, a bark doctor, a branch doctor, and on and on, instead of looking at the "root cause." Pun intended.

---

[11] Raju Kale and Roshan Deshmukh (2020)

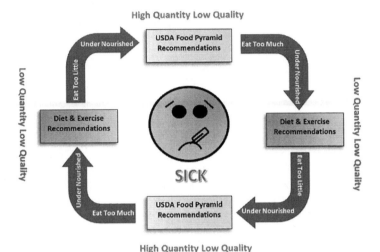

Fig 5: Vicious Cycle makes us all sick

If we stopped poisoning the tree, we could create an environment for the tree to thrive and exude the vitality it was designed to express. The tree would be strong, resilient, and vibrant. It would have the ability to bend but not break in bad weather. When the winds of life were howling and the rain was pounding on its leaves and limbs, it would stand strong grounded by its strong roots. The traditional model of systemic care weakens our roots and makes us extremely susceptible to any bad weather. Once again, the foundation on which our health and wellness recommendations are being based has nothing to do with creating vitality. If nothing else, it keeps us alive and more dependent on the very system that is creating the problem.[12]

---

[12] *If you would like to take an extraordinary and powerful deep dive into this idea, I'd recommend reading Dr. Gabor Maté's book, "The Myth of Normal" - Trauma, Illness, and Healing in a Toxic Culture. Gabor exposes the idea that what we have accepted as "normal" or "healthy" is actually illness, suffering, and pain.*

During the time Eve and I were not feeling all that well, we were consuming foods like salads, green veggies, grilled chicken, lean meat, whole grains, salmon, rice, and beans over 90 percent of the time. On paper, we couldn't have been eating a more "healthy" diet. The more we doubled down on this approach, the worse our symptoms got. We looked great, but we sure didn't feel great.

In Chapter 3, I will share with you the Vitality Principles for eating. The approach you will read about not only minimized, and in some cases eradicated our symptoms, it also gave us access to a level of energy and resiliency that we continue to enjoy today. I will also take you on a deeper dive into Eve's case study, where she was told at one point that she might not be able to have children due to hormonal issues, cysts, and other systemic complications. These issues were not only managed but completely overcome using the guidelines you will learn in this book.

Part III: The Problems with The Healthcare Paradigm for Mindset & Stress

The X-Factor

After learning such incredibly valuable information regarding proper movement, physical rehabilitation, and optimal nutrition, Eve and I decided to open our own clinic. It was our dream to open a clinic where we could empower individuals to experience a life of health and vitality they didn't realize was possible. After moving to Southern California, we opened our first clinic called Optimal Performance Institute, which we eventually renamed the Vitality Center. We offered corrective movement programming services helping individuals with every orthopedic injury you could think of, as well as nutritional courses and services. We had a thriving practice, often having a 3–4 week waiting list for people to get in to see us. Soon health professionals started asking us to teach them what we were doing. We eventually created and offered our own certifications in Corrective Movement Therapy and Nutritional Counseling. Over the course of the next six years, Eve and I were also blessed with two beautiful children. Things were cooking!

There was, however, one final piece of the puzzle that was still eluding me and would continue to stump me with some clients. This is what I referred to as the X-Factor. This "X-Factor" seemed to have a greater influence on someone's health and vitality than proper movement and good nutrition. The street name for this X-Factor was a mystical force called *stress*.

When working with some individuals, it often baffled me when I was unable to find anything significantly wrong with their biomechanics, meaning the way they moved, that correlated to the pain they were reporting. These same individuals also ate very well. I did, however, begin noticing a common denominator with these cases, and that was stress. These individuals seemed to be very stressed out. Either their overall state of stress was high or they were managing stressful events. Their symptoms seemed to directly correlate to their levels of stress. And I honestly didn't know what to say to them other than the standard things.

"Try not to be so stressed."

"Maybe a glass of wine would help."

"Have you tried a hot bath?"

These comments were not very helpful and many times left people feeling more frustrated and defeated.

Additionally, I was beyond stressed—trying to run a business, maintain a relationship with Eve, and be a father to my children. I was not doing an excellent job at any of these things. I kept things afloat, but none of them were thriving.

Colleagues told me to look into meditating. Some even sent me articles and meditations to do. I never did any of them. Who had time to meditate? I was way too busy.

That all changed one day after a week-long streak of leaving the house before Eve and the kids were awake and getting home after they were all asleep. I hadn't seen my family in over a week, and there was no sign of this pattern ending. Then it hit me—this is not OK! It was clear to me that this was going to lead to things that I definitely did not want—things like divorce, missing time with my kids, and getting sick.

It was time to do something about this so I started exploring all the personal development, psychological, and life coaching programs I came across. I read books, took courses, and even heavily dove into a specific personal development track of study for close to ten years.

Raised as a Roman Catholic and having a degree in psychology with a specialty in neuroscience, I had some basic concepts and belief structures around human behavior and morality and why people do what they do. The study of psychology and the brain has always fascinated me, so it was easy to dive back into the study.

I explored some of the basic principles and concepts of self-help, personal development, and psychology. The relative newness of these concepts and ideas was very interesting to me. Psychology as a study and the self-help industry are both less than 200 years old.[13] Samuel Smile's book, *Self-Help,* was published in 1859 and is considered to be the earliest and most successful self-help book. It is also how the industry

---

[13] McCloud Saul (2019)

got its name.[14] What existed before these categories emerged were philosophy and religious teachings.

Just as I did with movement and nutrition, I went all out in studying mindset, stress, and psychology. The place I took the deepest dive was a personal development organization that I helped build over about a seven-year period. When I got involved, it was a small organization run by an individual whom I perceived was able to really create incredible changes in people's lives. Many times I witnessed him help people reframe tragic events from their past and empower and free them from the enslavement of their circumstances. Working with individuals who had experienced traumatic events like rape, the death of children, and many other forms of terrible abuse, he meticulously walked them through a way to reexamine and reframe it, giving them a way to move forward. I watched him do this with people and thought to myself; "I *must learn how to support people in that way.*"

One of the most impactful things I learned at this time was how to manage that elusive X-Factor, stress. I was taught that stress was nothing more than how the mind perceived something and the emotions stirred up in the system were a result of this perspective. I am going to address the long-term limitations of this framework of stress later in this book, but at the time, it was helpful. During this period of time, I was learning how to become more aware of my emotions, how my thoughts reacted to them, and how to navigate through them. It was not only supportive to me at the time but also gave me a context to help support clients going through similar experiences. Additionally, I learned basic concepts to empower myself to drive and direct my life in ways I hadn't before. Simple concepts like

---

[14] Sinclair Marshall (2019)

- Naming what you want, not what you don't want
- Imagining the outcome before you fulfill the outcome
- Accepting your emotions
- Creating clearly defined benchmarks and goals

These basic concepts, which I have found to be in most self-help and personal development literature, were beneficial to get me out of my rut. I was then able to help many people by teaching these basic concepts to them.

My goal when working with someone is to make them more capable on their own and not need me. This was one of the most powerful things I learned from Lenny, my first mentor. When we started our physical rehabilitation clinic in Southern California, he told me that our goal was not to "put people on our 401K plan." It was his way of telling us we should not have our clients become so dependent on us that we were drawing money out of their accounts each month like a 401K plan. He said that our goal was to empower people by educating them about their bodies so they were self-sufficient. I loved that concept and positioning. It is something I will never forget and still practice today.

Throughout my time with this particular personal development organization, I became increasingly aware that many of the things I had learned through the years and wanted to incorporate into my work with the clients didn't fit in with the leader's vision. After a great deal of soul-searching, realizing we were no longer a good fit for each other. In October of 2021 I decided to step down from my position with this organization and resign.

Just as I found the prevailing wisdom in the diet and exercise world would not lead to a life of joyful vitality, I found that many of the general themes being used within the self-help and personal development industry created a level of dependency that was unacceptable to me. They are techniques and strategies that pit our mindset against our biology. This means that many of the common frameworks and approaches taught as common wisdom go directly against how our physiology and biology work. This creates one of two outcomes. The first outcome is a scenario where we will be "working on ourselves" forever because we can't overcome biology. An example of this is the idea that "you shouldn't care what people think." Over the years, I have heard people say they need to work on not caring what people think. Well, I can tell you those individuals are still working on it. They will be working on it forever because we are biologically wired to care what people think. It has been essential throughout human history to stay connected and to be part of a community or tribe to ensure our survival. If people don't like us, that is a problem that we should pay attention to and try to resolve. Otherwise, we will be on our own, and our chance of survival diminishes; thriving in life becomes impossible. It's not about not caring what people think about us; it's about learning how to channel that care, in a healthy way.

Working against our innate biology can also lead to the second outcome. This is complete dissociation from ourselves and these critical biological communications. Although it may be helpful to "not care about what people think about us" in the short term, it quickly has diminishing returns by causing us to disregard other biological communications that we depend on to stay connected. These individuals eventually begin to not trust themselves and, in the most severe cases, become completely disconnected from themselves. They become completely dependent on the system or individuals in which they are engaged to think for them.

I went through this journey when I was engaging in my deep dive into the personal development industry. I found a lot of benefits in getting involved in the work in the beginning. Because I give myself over completely to someone I believe I can trust, I learned the dangers of some of these concepts through first-hand experience. I got to the brink of completely dissociating from myself by disregarding all the intuitive communications that were screaming at me to get out. I am eternally grateful to the individuals who supported and guided me to trust myself in those moments, specifically my wife Eve and my dear friend Josh Guerrero.

I am super grateful I went through this process and extracted myself from the pull of dissociation. It has given me a much greater appreciation for the sacredness of the psyche, the value of psychology, and, most importantly, trust in the accuracy of how the human body communicates. It is invaluable when I am guiding other people through this process to ensure they are empowered.

Some of the concepts that I will be discussing that pit your mindset against your biology include

1. You shouldn't care what people think
2. When we are afraid, there is no real threat 99 percent of the time, so ignore it
3. Never take action when feeling negative emotions
4. You have "destructive patterns" that you need to eliminate
5. You shouldn't trust yourself when you are "emotional"
6. Happiness is a choice

I believe that human beings were designed to experience lives full of vitality, but I see that the way each system is set up does not empower us to create that life. Although there are places where the personal development system can be quite helpful, there is a strong tendency for it to keep us dependent on it. In this way it is similar to the traditional physical rehabilitative, systemic care, and nutrition industries.

The irony of this part of my journey is that I went into the world of self-help and personal development to manage my stress. Although it was helpful at times, especially in the beginning, the result was that it increased my stress to limits I could barely tolerate. A major concept I discuss in chapter seven is a new way to relate to stress and our emotions, so we are no longer managing them; we are partnering and leveraging them to move forward.

Although the journey was challenging, I am grateful for every experience because it showed me the importance of creating a new way to orient myself to health and wellness. The idea of "healthy" wasn't lining up with the standards that I was looking to experience in my life. I refused to settle for this idea of "healthy." It was evident that most approaches to maintaining a sound mind, body, and spirit were not very empowering and left people dependent on various modalities and systems.

In the following three chapters, I will share with you what I discovered throughout my journey. It is an entirely new paradigm that is anchored to principles of Vitality. These principles address the downfalls and limitations of the "health" paradigm. These principles are also intended to empower you to work interdependently with all the available resources and provide you with a solid foundation to make the most aligned decisions for your well-being. The Vitality Paradigm consists of three pillars, what I refer to as the Trilogy of Vitality. They include 1:Movement, 2:Systemic, and 3:Mindset, represented in Fig 6. If you were only to implement a few of the principles you will learn in this book, I guarantee it would give you access to more Vitality than you've ever known. Let's get started!

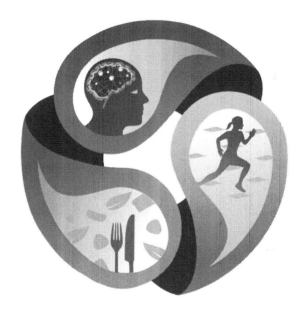

Fig 6: Trilogy of Vitality

TRILOGY OF VITALITY

PILLAR I: MOVEMENT

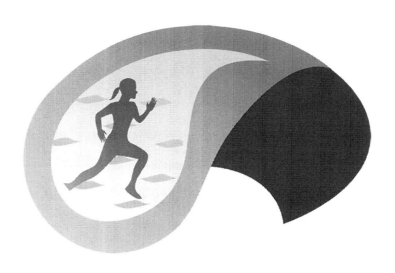

Chapter 3

STOP MOVING LIKE A DEAD PERSON

"It's Monday—chest and biceps day."
—*Every male that works out*

Understanding that the body was made to move and not to exercise is an essential concept and the place we are going to start. I have successfully rehabilitated thousands of individuals by simply teaching them the fundamentals of movement and reminding their bodies how they were designed to move.

After assessing the biomechanics of thousands of individuals, I can safely say that the people who were most likely to have forgotten how the body was designed to move were the personal trainers I worked with. At first, this doesn't seem to make any sense, but if you remember the orchestra analogy from Chapter 1, you will see how it can make perfect sense. They tended to move like robots, especially if trained in the traditional weight training model. This model applies what is called "split training." This is a form of programming that divides the body into parts. Back and tricep day, chest and biceps day, leg day, or days that focus on just the upper body and another on the lower body. This results in a disconnection between the parts of the body wherein one part of the body works in isolation of the other parts. To assess how well someone moved, I would have them perform fundamental movements like walking, squatting, and lunging. When personal trainers performed these motions, they moved as if they had to follow a set of rules like "spine straight," "draw in belly button," and "keep knee over the second toe." Their movements were rigid and segmented, not fluid and connected.

Most traditional personal training certifications, like the other areas of physical movement disciplines, are rooted in the application of cadaveric anatomy. The personal training and fitness industry is even *more* embedded in it because of its roots in bodybuilding. Bodybuilding had one objective - isolate areas and get them to grow.

This also meant making sure to burn a ton of calories (diet and exercise model) and focusing on shaping the specific areas of the body that weren't up to that individual's standards. The most common strategy is isolating an area and blasting it! Chest and biceps were the guys' favorite places to focus, and the ladies were all about the butt and abs. Guys never missed chest and bicep day, and women never missed butt and abs day. And I am not saying that this approach didn't work to grow mass and tighten up specific areas, but it also created a tremendous amount of dysfunction throughout the body.

As I mentioned in Chapter 1, isolating muscles and getting them to scream did accomplish the aesthetic objectives. And many of the personal trainers I worked with looked great but they were all in a lot of pain and in many cases, unable to perform some of the most basic movements. There was one personal trainer whom I knew who was the epitome of this reality . . . me.

My late teens and early twenties were some of my most extensive weight-lifting years. I worked out religiously and integrated every strength and fitness trick in the book—German volume training, super-sets, twenty-ones, heavy eccentric loading, 6:1 principle, compensatory acceleration, tempo training, and so on. There wasn't much I didn't try, and I got big and strong . . . unfortunately, it was only strong for the gym.

I got a job in my early twenties working on a construction crew framing houses. I was about 215 pounds and 8–10 percent body fat. I looked like a bodybuilder. When I walked onto that construction site, everyone looked at me and thought I would be able to move mountains. I would be able to tote plywood and lumber by the tons without breaking a sweat. Uh, yeah . . . not so much. There were guys half my size running circles around me. I could barely keep up for half a day. These guys would pick up a piece of plywood like it was nothing, fling it over the head, and almost jog to where they needed it, then skip back to the pile and do it again. I, however, worked through the pain and stiffness of getting into positions I wasn't used to, trying to press, carry, or drag a 4 x 8 foot piece of wood from the truck to the construction site. They could take 3–4 pieces to everyone I took. To say that was a humbling experience would be an understatement. It left me wondering how this could even be the case. I mean, I looked much stronger than they did. I had more muscle than they did. The difference was their strength was specific to their specific *life* needs and demands. My strength was created and designed to be executed in a gym.

This was one of my first and most valuable lessons regarding strength. I learned strength is only relative to the task. I was very strong on a bench in the gym, but that did not necessarily mean it carried over to vertical movements encountered on a construction site. And when I think about vitality, I think about being able to live my life to the fullest and having the ability to navigate all movements I'd encounter in life. This experience helped me realize I was only creating strength for artificial isolated movements that only take place in a gym.

When I had my clinic in Los Angeles, I posted this quote on the wall:

"Exercise is Optional, Movement is Mandatory."

I think of two contrasting paradigms, the movement paradigm and the exercise paradigm. The movement paradigm sees and acknowledges the enormous range of possibilities of movement and the infinite number of options that are available to a person. It also takes into consideration all the natural forces that influence and affect the body during movement. Natural forces like gravity, ground reaction forces, mass, and momentum. The interplay of these forces on the body dictate what the muscles are actually doing. The study of this interplay is called Chain Reaction Biomechanics™. This study and term was created by the founders of The Gray Institute, Gary Gray and Dave Tiberio. They are the fathers of functional anatomy and creators of Applied Functional Science. Applied Functional Science is the first to apply biological sciences of motion, reaction, proprioception, muscles, joints, mobility, and stability on the human body. That means that through this movement paradigm, any movement can be broken down to identify the specific action that each muscle in the body is doing. If you are a trainer, strength coach or work with human movement, the Gray Institute is the place to go to learn what the hamstrings are *actually* doing during movement, which is far more than flexing the knee.

On the other hand, the exercise paradigm creates "exercises" which make up a small subset of the infinite number of possible movements the body can perform (Fig

7). These exercises were created and designed using cadaveric anatomy. They are usually accompanied by many rules and guidelines and often isolate areas of the body and force them to work independently from the rest of the body. The exercise paradigm uses terms like agonist and antagonist, "this muscle is weak ", "this muscle is tight ". It holds, squeezes, and overall focuses on parts, not on the whole.

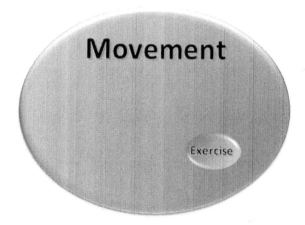

Fig 7: Exercise is a small subset of Movement

One of the most classic exercise paradigm applications gone wrong is the "cause of low back pain." The exercise paradigm will say most back pain is due to weak back and core muscles and tight hamstrings. The proposed remedy is to stretch the hamstrings, do dead bug core exercises (Fig 8), and back extensions. The approach is very myopic and isolates out the muscles that surround the spine and assumes that they are not performing their cadaveric anatomy functions. As you will see later in this chapter, this approach is extremely limited and inefficient. This certainly doesn't make all exercise paradigm applications bad, but it needs to be understood to avoid the downside.

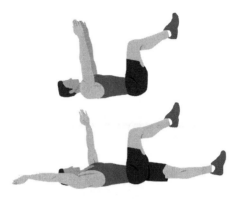

Fig 8: Dead Bug Core Exercise

Some common activities that fall into the category of "exercises" are bodybuilding, yoga, Pilates, spin, CrossFit, and sports. These are all variations of movements that have rules or specific tasks that are done repetitively to create a specific type of strength, capacity, or skill set. In the next chapter I will talk about how we integrate the movement paradigm into these types of activities and an athlete's programming.

When you look at the body through the movement paradigm, you will see an infinite amount of possibilities that exist. WIthin this range of possibilities, there are the foundational movement patterns that humans have been performing from the beginning of time. These include walking, squatting, lunging, reaching, pushing, pulling, and pressing. Now all these movements I just listed also have their "exercise version" counterparts. When I say squat, I am referring to a movement squat, not an exercise squat.

An exercise squat has a list of rules you must follow to execute correctly. The reason for the rules is to ensure you perform the movement safely. One of the key reasons why there is an inherent risk in the exercise squat is where the load is traditionally placed . . . on the upper back. When speaking strictly from a functional perspective, it is very inefficient to carry a load on the upper back. When you study cultures that carry heavy things, they carry them directly on top of their head. In certain tribes in East Africa, including the Luo, women can carry 70 percent of their body weight on their heads.[15] This is more efficient and much safer because the load is directly above our center of gravity, ensuring the load is evenly distributed and dispersed throughout the body, therefore not overloading any area.

Now I'm not suggesting you place the barbell on top of your head when squatting but because the squat exercise is not the best way to carry loads, we had to create rules to make it safe. These rules include eyes up, chest up, feet turned out, tightening the abdominals, and making sure your knees track over your second toe without them going past your toes. The reason for these rules is to ensure you don't hurt your back. If you were to look at the exercise squat (Fig 9) and ask where the only place on planet earth you would see someone performing this action, the answer would be the gym. This is a good sign that you are most likely in exercise land.

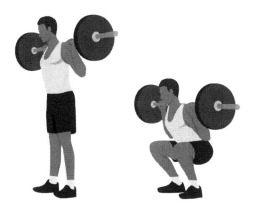

Fig 9: Exercise Squat

---

[15] Maloiy G et al. (1986),

A movement squat is very different and looks like something you are most likely already doing throughout your day. It looks like bending over to pick something up off the ground or sitting on a chair or toilet. (Fig 10) These actions are examples of movement squats and look very different from an exercise squat. Below is a case study that illustrates this idea.

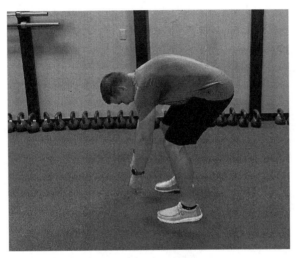

Fig 10. Movement Squat

THE TRILOGY & THE BIG ROCK

Before I dive into this first case study, I want to share my approach to assessing any client I work with who comes in with any physical ailment. I begin from a holistic perspective and do not make an assumption about why a person is presenting with their specific condition. I never assume a musculoskeletal injury is due to a biomechanical problem. I make sure to always look at what is happening systemically and mentally. I begin every evaluation by drawing a version of what you see in Fig 11, to educate the client about the ways these three factors contribute to their current condition.

TRILOGY OF VITALITY

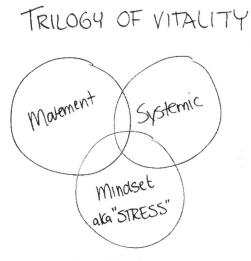

Fig 11: Trilogy of Vitality drawing from a client's initial assessment

These are the three factors that I refer to as the Trilogy of Vitality: Movement, Systemic, and Mindset, and what this entire book is about. The Movement component factors in how efficiently someone moves. The Systemic component looks at the variables impacting our system, like nutrition, sleep, hydration, and rest. The Mindset component factors in the impact of emotions, beliefs, attitudes, and other variables that influence overall stress. I assess all three of these components to get a big-picture view of a client's condition. Due to the infinite complexity and number of variables that could be contributing to someone's back hurting, I try to find in all my assessments something I call the "Big Rock". The Big Rock is the variable that is impacting a client's condition to the greatest degree. The first thing I assess is the

Global Big Rock. Meaning, is the client's current condition being influenced mostly by a biomechanical/movement dysfunction, a systemic dysfunction or an inability to manage stress. Once this is identified, then I focus on that specific component more directly to find the Big Rock within that specific component. For example if I suspect that the biomechanical component is the greatest contributor to their condition, I dive into that space to explore what biomechanical inefficiency is the Big Rock. You will see examples and references to this idea in each of the case studies throughout the book.

One of the main reasons I go through this thorough process is because of how easy it is to justify any dysfunction, found in any of the Trilogies of Vitality components, as the problem. Clients often ask me if I think their bed impacts their symptoms, their sneakers, the air they breathe, the water they drink, the electromagnetic waves in the air, pollution, or the fact that they sleep on the right side. My answer to all of these questions is 100 percent yes. All of these things are influencing their current condition. The more important question to ask is *which one* of these variables is having the greatest impact on your condition. If you address the big things, the little things tend to take care of themselves. The variable that I perceive to be having the greatest impact on a client's condition is the one I think of as the Big Rock. Once I identify the Big Rock, I start there.

One thing I believe is important for you to keep in mind when asking a professional to help you with your problem— is that they have an inherent bias and tendency to say the answer to your problem is what they specialize in. If you go to a podiatrist, inevitably you need orthotics. If you go to a chiropractor, then you need spinal alignment. If you go to a bodyworker, you need body work; if you go to an orthopedic surgeon, you need surgery. You may have heard the saying, if all you have is a hammer, everything looks like a nail. I have always loved Warren Buffet's advice, "Never ask a barber if you need a haircut."

Because of this inherent bias, I have attempted to create an evaluation framework that is intentionally objective that considers all the different variables within the Trilogy of Vitality. I also do my best during any assessment to make an effort to prove my initial assumptions wrong rather than try to prove them and convince myself they are right.

CASE STUDY

"I'm scheduled for surgery, but someone told me to come to see you first"

A young lady in her late thirties came to me because she suffered from debilitating low back pain that traveled down her leg. Her name was Anneliese, and she was in good physical health, exercised regularly, was very active, and took good care of herself overall. She had two small children, owned her own business, and was a full-time hairdresser. This back pain made it very difficult for her to do her job, not to mention tend to the needs of her two young children.

She came in as a last resort before what seemed like an inevitable surgery scheduled for later that month. She had already tried physical therapy, injections, and medications. None of them could address the problem. Someone gave her my name, in a desperate attempt to avoid surgery. She decided to come see if I could pull a rabbit out of my hat for her.

After spending some time going through her health history, I took her through a movement evaluation to assess her ability to perform the fundamental movements of walking, squatting, bending over, and reaching up -

essentially movements that I knew she performed every day. Knowing she was a mother, I knew the movements required were sometimes integrated and complex. I call being a mom an Olympic event. If you want to see complex movements, just watch a mom taking care of her children. I once saw a woman holding a squirming two-year-old in one arm and a large trash bag in the other. She somehow contorted her body to open a giant garbage can without dropping her two-year-old while calmly talking to her six and eight-year-old children in her periphery. Amazing!

As the evaluation began, I intended to find the Big Rock. I quickly observed that parts of her body were working as individual segments and they were not communicating with one another. It was as if they were all operating on their own islands, and it seemed like each segment was getting in the way of adjacent segments. Specifically, I noticed that anytime she moved, especially when squatting or lunging, her spine remained stiff and was not on the same page as her legs and hips. It was as if she were afraid to move it. This could be the Big Rock!

I taught her how to squat properly and explained that there were ways to squat that were not only safe for the low back but would make it stronger. The squat I demonstrated to her was the movement squat (Fig 10). This is a squat motion in which your eyes look to the ground, and the spine rounds. The key to executing this movement is ensuring the hips are the primary movers and take most of the load. For the hips to load properly, the pelvis must tip forward to flex the hip. From there, the spine must follow by flexing as well. When I suggested she try it, she immediately looked at me like I misspoke. Flexing her spine was exactly what the traditional model told her *not* to do. Now there is a time when you don't want to flex the spine, but I found that to only be the case in severe pathological conditions. I also knew as a hairdresser and mom that there was no way she wasn't going through that motion at times.

I encouraged her to try it and began to coach her through the movement. As she started performing the movement squat, after going through a moment of trepidation, she realized she was able to get all the way down without any pain at all. She even commented that it felt good on her back to be down there. After instructing her on how to use her strong legs to stand up, she was even more surprised when she could stand up without pain. But what really surprised her was that the movement felt good! I couldn't get her to stop doing it. She kept performing that movement squat repeatedly and had the biggest smile on her face.

Normally in these cases I would have had to do some bodywork to ensure the individual's soft tissues (muscles, tendons, ligaments, and fascia) were pliable enough for the movement to be performed properly - what I refer to as "clearing the runway." For Anneliese, her soft tissue runway was clear. It was just that she was caught in the exercise paradigm of movement and was never taught how to move properly for the tasks her body needed to do.

I never saw Anneliese for her back pain again after that session. She canceled her surgery and has had no low back pain in nearly four years.

The *NEW* Vitality Paradigm Part I: Movement

The Movement Principled Approach

One of my objectives at my clinic in Los Angeles was to produce at least a 50 percent improvement in three sessions or less. Anchoring to the movement principles allowed me to deliver on this objective.

As I have clearly stated, the traditional paradigm of exercise, fitness, and physical rehabilitation was based on cadaveric anatomy, which, when applied to a live, moving body, creates a ton of dysfunction throughout the body. Understanding how the body was designed to move is a critical first step to optimizing the body's performance and resiliency. Some key universal principles are important to understand when navigating movement. Not applying these principles will increase the likelihood of dysfunction and injury. Applying the principles below ensures that the body is being used in the way it was designed. This empowers you to partner with your body and maximize its potential.

5 Key Movement Paradigm Principles

1. The body always follows the path of least resistance
2. The body will sacrifice long-term health to survive at any moment
3. Strength and flexibility can only be measured relative to a task
4. The body moves in 3D from a macro and micro standpoint
5. Muscles lengthen before shortening to load (like rubber bands).

Movement Principle #1
Body Always Follows the Path of Least Resistance

The body's foundational mission and purpose is to stay alive and survive. The most basic need for survival is the ability to produce energy. When the cells can no longer produce ATP (energy), the body dies. This puts energy resources as a top priority and drives the body to conserve energy whenever possible—it certainly doesn't like wasting it.

And because of this, it always follows the path of least resistance. This is true from a movement standpoint but it also applies to other areas like the mind. If you have a strong belief about something, it is easier to continue to believe what you've always believed rather than to evolve and change that belief structure. The latter takes a lot of energy.

This principle can explain the reason for almost all back pain. Our society today is more sedentary than any other society known in the history of humankind. Our bodies were not designed to sit for hours and hours a day. One of the side effects of sitting is the tightness that manifests in our hips. Staying in a hip flexed position all day creates an adaptive shortening of the muscles in the front of the hip. This makes it difficult to extend the hips, which is necessary for standing and walking. When seated, the hips are in about ninety degrees of flexion (Fig 12a). When we get up from a chair and start walking around, we need approximately twenty degrees of hip extension to walk properly. (Fig 12b) This means that to go from sitting to standing we need the hips to make up a 110-degree difference! To make up for this difference, we need the muscles to be able to move 110 degrees from the moment we begin to stand to the first step we take. Due to the shortening of the anterior hip musculature when sitting, tightness and restriction in those muscles develop, making it difficult to get the required range of motion from the hips and stand up easily. This would account for the sound of effort people may make when getting up from a chair after sitting for a while. Due to this restriction in the hips, the body opts out of using the hips to walk properly and uses the low back to do the work instead. Although the back is able to tolerate this for some time, the body never considers the impact of using the spine to do the job of the hips long-term. It is choosing to use the back to work as the hips because it requires the least amount of energy in that moment and doesn't take into consideration the long term impacts. Which takes us to the next movement principle.

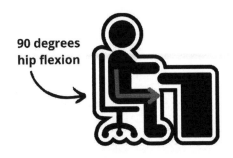

Fig 12a: Sitting, hip is flexed at 90 degrees

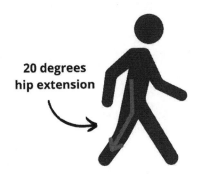

Fig 12b: Walking, hip needs to extend to 20 degrees

Movement Principle #2
The Body Will Sacrifice Long Term Health To Survive In Any Moment

As I mentioned, the body is first and foremost a survival machine. It has an incredible ability to adapt to a situation and keep going. This is a major asset that our bodies have, and because of this principle, many of us are still alive today.

Although these adaptations are crucial moment to moment, they can create many problems down the road that influence the quality of life. This can be seen in the example of the body using the back to walk, after sitting, instead of the hips. It gets the job done at that moment but costs down the road. You will see an example of this in the next case study. The body does not consider the long-term consequences of using the back as a hip. Asking a few segments of your spine to operate and do the job of your powerful hips will only deteriorate the spine over time. The amazing thing is the spine will do it for quite some time, but it is not sustainable and will eventually submit. I would say that most soft tissue injuries I have seen are a result of this principle. This makes keeping joints flexible and strong very important, which takes us to the third movement principle.

Movement Principle #3
Strength And Flexibility Can Only Be Measured Relative To A Task

When I hear people say they are strong or flexible or that a specific muscle is weak or tight, I always follow up with one key qualifying question: What position and motion was used to measure your strength or flexibility? One of the most common things I hear from clients is that their core is weak. This piqued my curiosity to learn exactly what they mean. I often ask them to tell me why they think that. They usually tell me about a specific exercise they cannot do, that they were told was a core exercise. For example, they can't hold a plank position for very long. The plank position is when you face the ground and hold yourself up on your forearms and toes, keeping the body nice and straight (Fig 13). Not being able to do this exercise very long means you are weak at one thing . . . being able to hold yourself in that position very long. To say that someone's core is weak because that can't be completed is a little extreme. The plank exercise is one of a possible million things your core musculature can do. It is mostly my back pain clients that come to me and tell me their problem is that their core is weak and that they have been trying to strengthen their core doing these types of exercises. This is exactly why they are at the point of seeking out my help—it doesn't work.

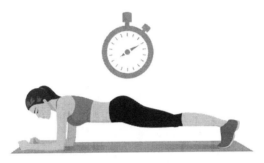

FIg 13: Plank Exercise

There is no exercise or test that universally defines weakness, strength, tightness, or flexibility. The only thing any exercise does is simply tell us a story about that specific position and motion. When you test someone's ability to stand and touch their toes, you are testing someone's ability to stand and touch their toes . . . that's it. This is very important because I have seen people prescribed entire protocols to address their tightness or weakness, which was never specifically defined, and then given some canned protocol of stretching or strengthening that has no carryover to what they need.

In the case of Annelise, the type of therapy she was receiving was exactly this. She was told her back and core were weak, and her hamstrings were too tight. She was then given exercises to strengthen her back and core and stretches for her hamstrings like the ones in Fig 14. These back extensions and variety of core exercises may look familiar to some of you. What we needed to do instead is to identify the specific motion and position the pain was associated with and then address the inefficiencies of the biomechanics in those specific positions and motions. When someone has back pain, we want to ask in what position and in what motion does the pain occur? This allows us to be much more targeted and specific to each individual's needs. Someone with pain in the back when sitting and rotating to the right should have a very different rehab program than someone with pain in their back when bending over.

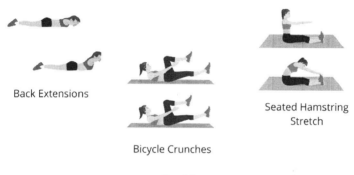

Back Extensions

Bicycle Crunches

Seated Hamstring Stretch

Fig 14

The number of people with whom I've worked with who have come to me with back pain and were told their core and back are weak, or their hamstrings or psoas (a hip flexor muscle located in the front of the hips) is tight, has to be in the hundreds if not thousands. The "weakness" or "tightness" found in these isolated muscles are the result of the dysfunction of the movement strategies, they are not the cause. One thing I emphasize with the practitioners I have trained is to stop being muscle specific with their evaluation and start being movement specific. Don't ask what muscle is the problem; focus on what movement is the problem.

Movement Principle #4
The Body Moves in Three Dimensions
(Macro and Micro)

When evaluating movement, we must consider that we are three-dimensional creatures. Our body is designed to move in three dimensions. The three dimensions are sagittal, frontal, and horizontal planes. (Fig 15) Sagittal is a front-to-back motion, frontal is a side-to-side motion, and horizontal is a rotational motion. The body moves through these dimensions at a macro level and at a micro level. An example of a macro sagittal plane motion is walking in a straight line, forward or backward. Sliding side to side like a defensive player in basketball is a frontal plane motion, and swinging a golf club would be more of a horizontal plane motion.

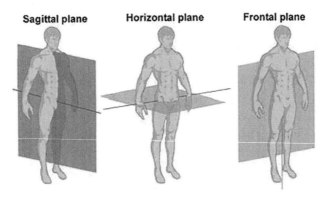

Sagittal plane   Horizontal plane   Frontal plane

Fig 15: Three Planes of Motion[16]

Not only does our body move in these three dimensions globally, but it also moves in three dimensions on a micro level. For example, if you look at the hip joint, where the head of the femur meets the cup of the pelvis called the

---

[16] Walden Michael (2021)

acetabulum, you will notice that this joint moves in three dimensions. (Fig 16) The hip can flex and extend in the sagittal plane, abduct and adduct in the frontal plane, and internally and externally rotate in the horizontal plane. As a matter of fact, every joint in the body can move in all three dimensions. What is even more fascinating is if you were to watch a human walk from a bird's eye view under an X-ray, you would see every single joint in the body working together, in synchronous coherence, in all three planes of motion, to produce the result of walking forward. It is just like a finely tuned and trained orchestra making beautiful music. This is why it is critical to ensure that any stretching or strengthening program addresses all three planes of motion. Most of the traditional stretching and strengthening exercises are uni-dimensional in their approach. Examples of this are illustrated in figure 17, with the classic hamstring stretch and the traditional lunge exercise.

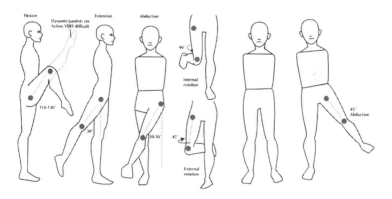

Fig 16: Motions of the Hip Joint

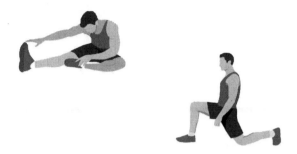

Fig 17: One Dimensional Hamstring Stretch & Lunge

**Movement Principle #5
Muscles Lengthen Before They Shorten**

The best way to think about muscles is like super sophisticated rubber bands. The key feature of a rubber band is that, in order to access its potential power and force, you must lengthen it first. You can't shoot a rubber band across the room unless you pull it back first. This is how you want to think about your muscles. To access the power of your musculature, you must be able to lengthen the muscle. This is why every motion starts with the opposing motion. Every motion up starts with a motion down. Try to jump straight up in the air without going down to the ground first—not possible.

If you look at traditional exercises, the focus on building strength is the opposite of how muscles work. The traditional emphasis is always put on the shortening, squeezing, and contraction of the muscle. You will see trainers in gyms around the country cuing their clients to squeeze their muscles, hold them, and contract them harder. This is an example of taking a tuba from an orchestra, isolating it, and asking it to play as loudly as possible, wondering why it doesn't sound like music. Isolating and emphasizing the shortening of individual muscles, is what creates all the "noise" and dysfunction in the body.

Application of The Movement Principles: Stretching

One of the areas where I find a lot of confusion and poor application is in the space of stretching. I have identified two reasons to stretch:

1. To warm up the body for a specific activity
2. To create new motion at a joint

If you feel tight and want to become more flexible, ask yourself what specifically you want to be flexible for. If it is for the normal activities of daily living, then your stretch program should look like the activities of your daily living. If most of your day is upright and on your feet, you want to ensure your stretches are not all taking place on the ground. Make sure that you are doing stretches where you are standing. You should also ask yourself when you are doing a movement or stretch if it resembles anything you do in your daily routine. If you want to feel more flexible to play tennis or golf, then you want your stretch and warm-up routine to look similar to tennis or golf.

On the other hand, if you find a major restriction in a joint or region of the body during these stretches and movements, you must learn how to do "sniper stretching." Sniper stretching is a technique that I use to help people create new motion at joints and regions throughout their bodies. It ensures that the motion is being created where intended—it has to be very targeted, like a sniper. Because the body always follows the path of least resistance, we have to be extremely calculated when trying to create new motion at a joint because we are essentially attempting to go into a path that has great resistance and restriction.

If we are not diligent in our application, the body will start to pick up a range of motion at adjacent joints that are already moving too much. This can worsen the situation, leading to injury. In figure 18, I am demonstrating what happens when a common movement, intended to stretch the hips, is done improperly. You will see that I am getting way too much motion in my spine which is an indication that I am not getting enough motion from my hips. This is similar to the earlier example of what happens when we sit too long. This is a classic example of how stretching can cause more harm than good.

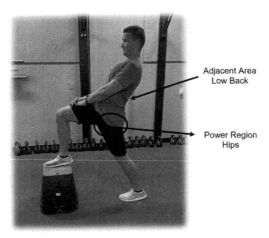

Adjacent Area
Low Back

Power Region
Hips

Fig 18: The improper way to stretch the hips due to excessive motion in the lumbar spine

Another important thing to note are two reasons a muscle in the body can present as tight. When there is tightness or restriction in a muscle or region of the body, it is important to distinguish if the restriction or tightness is there because it is protecting something or if it is mechanically stuck. Protective tightening is when muscles are tight because they are protecting something that is damaged or compromised, like nerve damage, torn or ruptured soft tissues, or an unstable joint. The last thing you want to do is stretch or mobilize an area that is protectively tightening. Mechanical tightness is when muscles have been tight and restricted for so long that they form high amounts of scar tissue and become stuck. In these cases, targeted stretching and bodywork are necessary to mobilize the area. In the case study below, I share when I learned the difference between protective tightening and mechanical tightness.

CASE STUDY

"I don't think this is a good idea."

In my earlier years of learning and applying these principles, I had a woman in her late sixties named Alana come to see me for some chronic back pain issues. She and her husband David were super active. One of the things she and her husband loved to do was get in their RV and travel around the country. Her husband was retired military where he had specialized in extracting wounded soldiers from the fields of combat - he had many injuries. I also worked with him. To say they were going to live their lives the way they wanted despite the state of their bodies was an understatement. They were pursuing life in inspiring ways. Alana was one of those clients I wished I had fifty of. She was collaborative, had a great attitude, understood her situation, and was ready to find root causes. She was also witty, sarcastic, and super smart. She even taught me some great Yiddish words like "schmatta." That's what she called the top I asked her to wear while I worked on her back. We had a lot of good laughs. Alana had navigated a lot of physical and emotional situations in her life. She had some significant structural limitations that we needed to work around, like severe deterioration of regions of her spine. She also challenged me with many questions asking me why I was doing what I was doing and wanting to understand her body. I love clients like this—ones that don't just accept what I'm saying because I'm the professional but ask great questions and want to be empowered with knowledge.

After performing a biomechanical movement assessment that included a comprehensive gait (walk) assessment, a series of squatting and lunging movements, and a thorough table assessment, I identified significant mechanical tightness in her hips, especially the right hip; this was her Big Rock. I treated her hips by doing precise soft tissue bodywork techniques and a variety of sniper stretches to increase the hips' ability, specifically her right hip, to internally rotate more efficiently. After clearing the soft tissue runways, I taught her how to integrate this new hip motion into the foundational movement patterns. I focused mostly on walking, squatting, and lunging since those were the primary movements in her extremely active life. She was extremely active. After working with Alana for a few weeks, her back pain was becoming much less frequent, and when it was present, it wasn't debilitating—she was overall doing much better.

Alana and her husband tended to push their thresholds which got them into trouble at times. The upside was I helped them be in less pain and be more capable. The downside was they were in less pain and more capable. This meant they *could* push their boundaries and say, "No worries, Matt will straighten us out." Well, one day Alana came to see me because her back was spasming—they overdid it on an intense hiking and camping trip. She asked me if I could do a technique on her back that she felt would be helpful. It was a technique I used to decompress the back through a fascial soft tissue mobilization. My instincts told me this was a bad idea, and I told her I thought it would make it worse if I did that. I explained that when muscles go into spasm, they are protectively tightening because of a potential instability in the region. Essentially, that area is being asked to move too much relative to its ability. So I convinced her that I should work on her hips and not touch her back . . . until the end of the session. She asked again to do the technique on her back, believing it would help. Ultimately, I gave in. After performing the technique on her back, she immediately felt relief. When she got off my table, her back went into severe spasm, and she dropped to the ground. I felt terrible! I knew I shouldn't have gone against my better judgment. It was not a good scene. But true to form, Alana said, "You were right, Matt; this is not your fault. I should have listened to you. No worries. I'll just crawl out of your office and get David to pick me up and load me into the truck. I'll be fine. See you next week!" And she did. This was when I learned the importance of assessing protective tightening versus mechanical tightness.

Now let's assume that a client was presenting with a mechanical tightness. In this case, very specific and targeted soft tissue work and stretching would apply, like the work I did on Alana's hips. I emphasize targeted and precise stretching because we need to manage the reality the body is always following the path of least resistance. We have to remember that the body doesn't want to go against the resistance of the shortened soft tissues, even if it means injury in the future.

When stretching the body, it is important to know the objective. You are either stretching to create a new range of motion or to gain access to the motion you have. The former requires you to be more mindful because of the risk associated with stretching a protectively tight muscle. For the latter, it is necessary to be clear about what activity you are preparing the body to perform so your stretch protocol looks similar to that activity. For example, if you are stretching your body before running and your stretch protocol is on the floor, you are not preparing it for running because running doesn't take place on the floor.

The last thing to note when stretching is to ensure you are stretching in all three dimensions. Giving the muscles of the body access to lengthen in all three dimensions gives the body access to all of its potential power.

Tom Brady, future Football Hall of Famer and the G.O.A.T. has played over twenty years at an elite level in the most unforgiving sport—football. In this sport, the average career is slightly over three years. One of the main reasons he has accomplished this is his approach to training his body. He spends the majority of his training taking care of his soft tissues with massage, bodywork, and stretching protocols that look like the tasks he performs. If you look at his training program TB12™, there is very little to no heavy weight training and most of his movements look like football movements.

Through applying these five movement principles in my twenty years of working with thousands of individuals, I have identified some essential areas that must be addressed in order to sustain optimal performance over time. I call these areas the Power Regions.

The Power Regions of the Body

As I mentioned earlier, the body moves through three primary dimensions, sagittal, horizontal, and frontal. What is interesting about these three planes of motion is their orientation to gravity. One of the three planes has a unique orientation to gravity. As illustrated in figure 19, gravity directly lines up with the sagittal and frontal planes. This means that it directly opposes those two planes. An example of a sagittal plane motion that opposes gravity would be lifting your arm directly in front of you. A frontal plane example would be lifting your arm to the side. If you held your arms in either of these positions, they would eventually fatigue because of the weight of gravity. The horizontal plane, on the other hand, does not oppose gravity. If you were to stand up and turn your hips to the right and to the left, gravity does not oppose that motion. Any limitation you would feel would be tightness in your soft tissues.

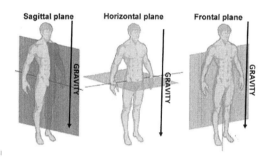

Fig 19: When looking at the force of gravity coming straight down, you will see that the horizontal plane of motion is the only one not in the plane of gravity and therefore does not oppose the force.

So why is this significant? It is significant because the body will always favor loading itself in the horizontal plane because there is no opposing force or resistance it needs to overcome. It is the path of least resistance. What it also does is allows the muscles to easily lengthen and load (like a rubber band) in the "free plane" to set it up to effectively unload in the two planes (sagittal and frontal), that oppose gravity. Quite brilliant, if you ask me.

Now, if that was too much technical jargon and I lost you, don't worry; it's not essential to understand it to that depth. What is important to understand is that the body is designed to load in the horizontal plane. It is where the system operates at its optimal level. Every joint and muscle can move in three planes (movement principle 4). That being said, it is important to note that each joint or region of the body has a dominant plane of motion in which it operates. A great example is the knee joint—although it can move in all three planes, it is predominantly a sagittal plane joint (hinge joint) - meaning it bends really well, but is limited in rotation and lateral motion. There are also regions of the body that specialize or are dominant in certain planes of motion. An example of this is the lumbar spine. The lumbar spine is made up of five vertebral bodies and the sacrum. These are called L5, L4, L3, L2, L1, and S1, where the "L" stands for lumbar and "S" stands for sacrum. (Fig 20)

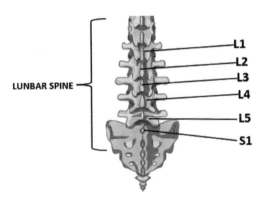

Fig 20: Lumbar Spine

The lumbar spine was designed to move primarily forward and backward (sagittal plane) and side to side (frontal plane). It is not so efficient at rotating in the horizontal plane. If you summated the rotational ability of each segment in this region, it would only equate to about thirteen degrees of rotation. This is very little and cannot be seen with the naked eye. What is impressive about the body, is that if there is a joint or region that is limited in one plane of motion, there will be a neighboring joint(s) that dominates in that plane of motion. In the cases of the lumbar spine and the knee, both having significant limitations in their ability to rotate, they have one of the most robust rotating joints living right next door—the hips. For this reason, the hips are a *joint* that I refer to as a Power Region.

The Power Regions are joints or regions of the body that have the greatest ability to rotate and, therefore, the greatest ability to take on the bulk of the forces and distribute them safely. The regions with the greatest gross rotational ability are the foot and ankle complex, the hip complex, and the thoracic spine. The thoracic spine consists of twelve vertebral bodies between the lumbar and cervical spine. It is also the part of the spine where the ribcage attaches (Fig 21).

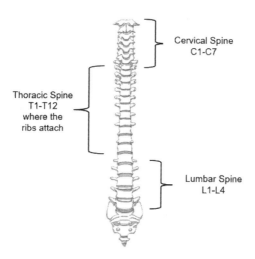

Cervical Spine
C1-C7

Thoracic Spine
T1-T12
where the
ribs attach

Lumbar Spine
L1-L4

*Fig 21: Three regions of the spine:
cervical, thoracic, and lumbar*

Looking at the structure of the thoracic spine versus the lumbar spine segments, you will see a significant structural difference. The lumbar spine stacks the vertebrae on top of each other in an overlapping manner creating facet joints (Fig 21a). These facet joints have the lumbar segments interlocked, creating more ability to bear load and stabilize but sacrifices their ability to rotate. When you compare the vertebral bodies of the thoracic region, you will notice a very different structure. The thoracic vertebrae are sitting more on top of one another, allowing them to rotate on each other much easier (Fig 21b). This is what makes the thoracic spine *region* a Power Region.

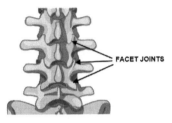 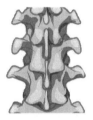

21a. Lumbar Vertebrae   21b. Thoracic Vertebrae

Fig 21a/21b: Notice that the structure of the thoracic vertebral segments is very different than the structure of the lumbar vertebral segments allowing them to rotate on top of one another more easily

Who The Power Regions are Protecting

It's not a coincidence that the areas that surround the Power Regions are usually the most problematic areas - the cervical spine, glenohumeral joint (shoulder), low back, and knees. These areas are highly susceptible to being asked to rotate too much when the power regions are not doing their job, which creates wear and tear, leading to injury. We saw an example of this in the case study with Alana. Her spine had degenerative changes over time, and a significant reason for the degeneration was the inability of her hips to distribute forces away from her spine. She was an administrative assistant for over thirty years, so she did a ton of sitting, which substantially locked up her hips. Over time, the lack of motion in her hips started to chew away at her spine. Although there isn't much one can do to reverse degeneration in the spine, there is a lot you can do to slow down to prevent further degeneration.

Here is an overview of the Power Regions & their susceptible neighboring joints: (Fig 22)

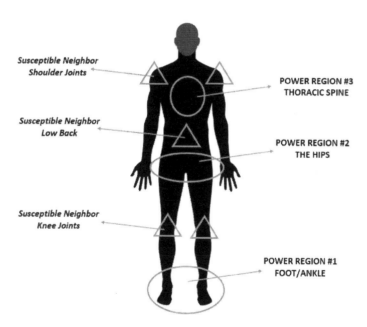

Fig 22: Power Regions and their neighboring joints that are susceptible to over rotating

Power Region #1: Foot and Ankle Complex

The Power Region that is by far the most dynamic, intricate, and complex is the foot and ankle complex. Twenty-six bones, thirty-three joints, and twenty-nine muscles make up this region. The foot and ankle complex play an essential and paradoxical role in movement. Its job is to act like a soft pillar for landing and be a stable platform to push off from. It does these two actions by performing the motion of pronation (absorbing load) and supination (unloading). These two actions also convert the forces of gravity and ground reaction forces to move up and down the kinetic chain efficiently.

Foot and Ankle as Shock Absorber and Stable Propeller

When our foot hits the ground, it unlocks and splays itself out to absorb the convergence of the two opposing forces, gravity and the ground reaction. As it collapses, it performs a spiraling inward motion into the ground (pronation). This spiraling internal motion into the ground is sent up the kinetic chain, lengthening and loading the musculature of the posterior chain - specifically the calf, hamstring, and hip complex. This action is the *key* to turning on and activating the musculature of the glutes to ensure the hips are participating in movements. This is why the foot is considered the switch that turns on the butt.

This leads me to an important point. So many people have come to me over the years and told me their "butt doesn't fire". They also share that they are working on getting it to fire by doing exercises like clams or bridges. I hope you are starting to see why these exercises are not practical for a variety of reasons. For one it isolates the muscles and asks it to scream and second it doesn't take into consideration the foot's relationship with the hips. Think of the foot like a light switch on your wall. If you were to walk into a room in your house with the lights off, I'd imagine you would go to the light switch first. You wouldn't change the bulb to a higher wattage hoping that a higher watt bulb would magically turn on the light. Changing the light bulb to a higher wattage is analogous to doing isolated butt squeezing exercises, like clams and bridges, to try to turn on the butt. If you want to activate and turn on the glutes, you need to make sure the switch to the butt—the foot and ankle complex—is working.

Once the foot can absorb the load and activate the glutes, it now has to completely reverse its formation and go through the motion of supination, become rigid by locking itself up so the glutes can unload the force of propulsion and the body has a stable propeller from which to push off. (Fig 23) The foot and ankle complex must be able to perform both of these motions efficiently.

RIGHT FOOT

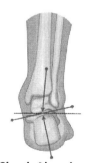
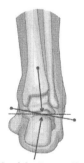

Shock Absorber
Right foot pronating to
absorb load in walking

Stable Propeller
Right foot supinating to create
stable platform for push off

Fig 23: The dynamic role the foot and ankle play in movement

Two Key Areas of the Foot and Ankle Complex

There are two major joints that are important to acknowledge and understand within the foot and ankle complex. The two joints are the talocrural joint and the subtalar joint. Not only do each of these joints play important roles individually, but they also play a crucial role when their motions are combined. The talocrural joint is where the sagittal plane motion takes place—what is referred to as plantar flexion and dorsiflexion of the foot and ankle. The subtalar joint is a saddle joint and gives the foot and ankle the ability to move in the frontal plane or from side to side, like the saddle of a horse. The combination of these two joint motions creates the rotational capacity of the region, which is pronation and supination. The ability of these two joints to play their roles interdependently and convert the rotational loads through the body makes this a Power Region.

An exercise that you can try that demonstrates the rotational capacity of your foot and ankle complex is a standing rotational movement. Stand barefoot on the ground with feet pointed straight and shoulder-width apart. Place your arms straight out in front of you at about chest height. Now rotate your arms as far to the left as you can. Notice that the arch of your right foot has flattened or, at the very least, is moving toward the floor. You will also notice that the arch of your left foot is more arched, and you are on the outside of the left foot. Now, if you take your arms and rotate them all the way to the right, you should experience a complete reversal of this motion. Your left arch should now be flattening, and your right arch should be rising. As you move the arms back and forth, you will start to feel and connect to all the rotation in your foot and ankle complex. If you didn't experience this, you will want to go through the Power Region Program that I put together for you in the next chapter - because that's a problem.

Power Region #2: Hip Joint

The hip joint is one of the most powerful joints in the body. It is where the femur bone and the pelvis meet. The head of the femur sits in the area of the pelvis called the acetabulum. (Fig 24) Because the femur is round and sits in a cup-like area of the pelvis, it has a tremendous ability to rotate, giving it an extensive range of motion.

HIP JOINT

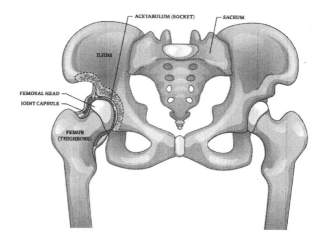

Fig 24: Hip joint

As a ball and socket joint, the hip has the capacity to move significantly in all three dimensions. The sagittal plane's full range of motion is approximately 160 degrees—30 degrees of extension and 130 degrees of flexion. In the frontal plane, it has a total range of motion of 75 degrees, 45 degrees of abduction, and 30 degrees of adduction. And in the horizontal plane, it has a total range of motion of 85 degrees, 45 degrees of external rotation, and 40 degrees of internal rotation. (Fig 25)

Because of all this available motion, the muscles and ligaments surrounding the hip joint are some of the largest and strongest in the body. There are a total of twenty-one muscles that cross the hip joint. There aren't many movements that humans perform that don't require hip involvement at some level. Whether you are crawling on the ground, walking, squatting, lunging, sitting, bending over, or rolling over, the hips play a role. For all these reasons, this is the second power region of the body.

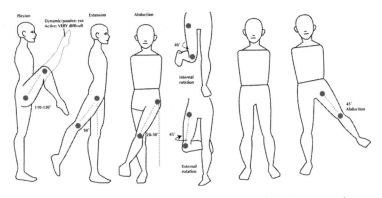

Fig 25: All the available range of motion of the hip complex

Power Region #3: Thoracic Spine
(and Scapula-Thoracic Joint)

The third power region is the thoracic spine. The thoracic spine is the other region of the body where we have access to a significant amount of rotation. The thoracic spine consists of twelve vertebral bodies. As you may recall, the significance of these vertebral bodies is the unique way they are structured relative to other parts of the spine. Their structure enables them to rotate to a much higher degree, especially when compared to the lumbar spine. (Fig 21a/b)

Each thoracic vertebral body can rotate about three degrees to the right and three degrees to the left. When you summate the rotational ability of these 12 segments, as a unit it provides 30–35 degrees of rotation in each direction. This gives the thoracic spine the ability to move upward of 70 degrees total. Comparatively, the lumbar spine's gross rotational ability is about twenty-five degrees.

The thoracic spine is also where the ribs originate. This is important because the four primary abdominal muscles insert to the ribcage: internal and external obliques, rectus abdominis, and transversus abdominis.(Fig 26) Therefore, in order to lengthen, to properly load the abdominals, it is essential the thoracic spine is able to rotate sequentially so that the ribs are able to dissociate from the pelvis and properly lengthen the abdominals. Lengthening these muscles in the horizontal (rotational) plane produces a tremendous amount of potential power and creates stability through the core to protect the lumbar spine.

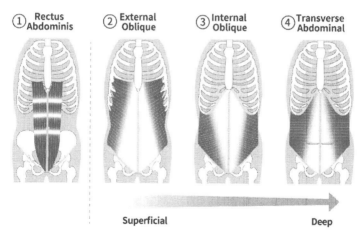

Fig 26: Key abdominal musculature insert on the ribcage

The other significant region that works closely with the thoracic spine is the scapula-thoracic joint. (Fig 27) This is where the shoulder blade sits on the ribcage. It is called a floating joint because it has no bony attachment to the ribcage. It floats on the upper posterior portion of the ribcage and plays an integral role in proper thoracic and shoulder motion.

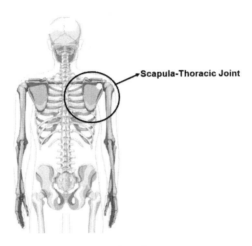

Scapula-Thoracic Joint

Fig 27: Scapula-Thoracic Joint

As I mentioned earlier, the neighboring areas of the Power Regions are most susceptible to injury. This is why it is not a coincidence that they are where the most common orthopedic injuries take place (Fig 28). Torn meniscus (knee), carpal tunnel syndrome (wrist), torn rotator cuff (shoulder), torn ACL (knee), and tennis elbow are some of the most common orthopedic injuries. The best way to avoid these injuries and rehabilitate these injries and many others, is to address the Power Regions.

One of the main reasons I can throw a baseball today is because I learned how to leverage my Power Regions to throw. Learning how to properly ground myself through my foot and ankle complex, integrate my hips and thoracic spine into the throwing motion was a game changer. I have worked with a ton of volleyball players, pitchers, and tennis players who all came in with a variety of arm and shoulder injuries. The way I rehabbed them was by giving them access to their power regions and then teaching them how to leverage and integrate the power regions to take the unnecessary stresses off their extremities. Not only did this eliminate their pain, but integrating the power regions efficiently into the complex movements like throwing, serving, or spiking a volleyball vastly improved their power, speed, and overall performance.

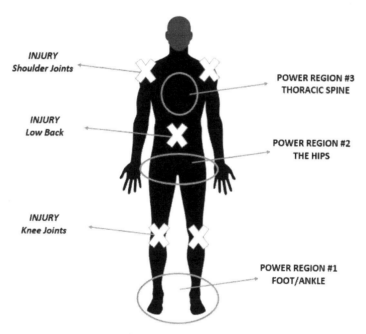

INJURY
Shoulder Joints

INJURY
Low Back

INJURY
Knee Joints

POWER REGION #3
THORACIC SPINE

POWER REGION #2
THE HIPS

POWER REGION #1
FOOT/ANKLE

Fig 28: Joints in between and adjacent to the Power Regions are more susceptible to injury

One of the best ways to keep the body in optimal condition is to make sure you keep the access to your Power

Regions open and ready for action. In the next chapter, I share the Vitality Movement Framework that I have developed to not only rehabilitate injuries, but to increase optimal levels of performance. You will also get access to a program that you can use to ensure your Power Regions are in optimal condition for whatever activities your specific lifestyle demands.

Chapter 4

THE VITALITY FRAMEWORK
FOR MOVEMENT

At my clinic in Los Angeles, I created a framework to assess clients and design their treatment programs. I trained the clinicians who worked in my practice and practitioners from all over the country to use this method. Many continue to leverage these philosophies and have thriving practices to this day. The framework is illustrated below in Figure 29.

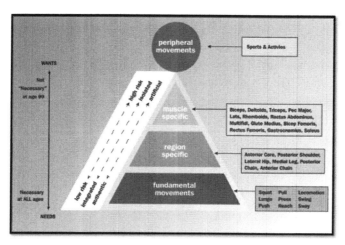

Fig 29: The Vitality Movement Framework

As you can see, everything was based on fundamental movements. This was the foundation of the approach—always working to and from the improvement of a fundamental movement pattern listed in the diagram: squat, lunge, push, pull, press, reach, locomotion, swing, and sway. This was where every assessment began. We always wanted to assess the body's ability to move as a whole entity, regardless of the client's condition.

After assessing global movement patterns we then progressed to the region specific assessments. The region we assessed was determined by what we saw in the fundamental movements. If we saw what we suspected to be a limitation in the hip region when someone was walking, we assessed the hip region more specifically. Lastly, if necessary, we assessed the relevant muscles by either isolating them with muscle tests or palpating the tissues manually.

The reason for this global approach was to keep us connected to the fundamental movement we were trying to improve. Because of the complexity of each part of the body, when we needed to address a specific part, we needed the reference point of the fundamental movement to ensure we didn't get lost in the parts. The diagram you see is the exact diagram posted in my clinic. It helped us remember why we were doing what we were doing and how we were doing it.

The rest of what you see in the diagram are also aspects of our overall philosophy. Running along the left side of the overall triangle you will notice three continuums listed — authentic to artificial, integrated to isolated, and low risk to high risk. This is to educate clients that the more muscle specific the technique or exercise is, the more artificial, isolated, and higher risk it is. We felt it was important for our clients to know the facts so they could better navigate their movement and exercise selection. On the flip side, the closer the technique or exercise was to the fundamental movements, the more authentic, integrated, and low risk it would be.

As an example, if you were to compare the seated dumbbell bicep curl with an anterior lunge and a reach to the floor, you could easily determine which exercise, if done repetitively, would lead to wear and tear faster and have a higher risk of injury. This is assuming both exercises were being executed properly (Fig. 30). The elbow joint was not designed to work in isolation under load over and over again, as it does in a seated dumbbell curl. However, an anterior lunge with a reach to the ground is essentially stepping forward and picking something up, which the human body has been doing since the beginning of time.

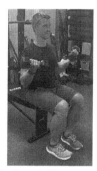
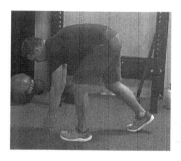

Isolated Bicep Curl   Integrated Anterior Lunge with Reach

Fig 30: Isolated bicep curl vs. an integrated anterior lunge with reach.

This is also where the final plumb line on the left of the diagram, NEEDS to WANTS, comes into play. This was to reinforce our NEED to be able to do the fundamental movements for our entire life, while our engagement in the more specific and complex movements, like bicep curls and the ones represented by the giant ball on the top of the triangle, are things we may WANT to be involved in.

The giant ball on the top of the pyramid is labeled *peripheral movements*. This is where sports and activities belong. We included this for our athletes. Because sports and activities are made of movements that are repetitive and specific to the tasks of the sport, there is more inherent risk of injury. The problem with many of the athletes we worked with was that most of them only engaged in the sport they played and performed muscle-specific exercises. FOr example, a basketball player, played basketball and did muscle specific exercises like traditional bench pressing, back squatting, shoulder presses, and bicep curls. This is why so many of the athletes were injured. We taught and trained our athletes to build a strong and stable movement foundation by training three dimensional movement patterns that incorporated the entire muscle system, teaching it to work as an integrated unit. This strong foundation made it easier to balance the peripheral movement ball on top of the triangle.

Based on this overall framework I created four phases that I used to guide people through the rehabilitation process. The four phases were:

1. Remodel
2. Reprogram
3. Condition
4. Enhance

The remodel-reprogram-condition-enhance system takes into account the movement paradigm principles and the above framework. Below is a program I created to facilitate proper mobility, stability, and strength in the Power Regions that translate to everyday activity. You can access the accompanying videos for each of the exercises in the table below by going to www.*healthtovitality.com/resources*

POWER REGIONS PROGRAM

REGION	REMODEL Ball or Foam Rolling	REPROGRAM	CONDITION	ENHANCE
Foot-Ankle Complex	Bottom of foot Peroneals Calf complex	Standing 3D Foot & Ankle Mobilization	Dynamic Foot & Ankle Mobilization	Standing 3D Balance Foot Reach
Hip Complex	Glutes Front of Hip Quadriceps Side of Hip	Level I: Standing 3D Hip Mobilization / Level II: Kneeling 3D Hip Mobilization	Level I: 3D Walking / Level II: 3D Step ups	3D Lunge Matrix / 3D Uncommon Lunge Matrix
Scapula-Thoracic Complex	Lats Chest Thoracic Mobes Thoracic Matrix	Standing Two Arm Reach Stretch Matrix	Standing Alternate 3D Press Matrix	Single Leg Alternating 3D Press Matrix

Go to www.healthtovitality.com/resources to access the accompanying videos,

where I walk you through each of the three Power Regions.

The Remodel, Reprogram, Condition, and Enhance Approach to Programming

PHASE I: Remodel

The first step in the process is the remodeling phase. This phase addresses any mechanical tightness or restrictions. These are the limitations in the soft tissues that may be restricting or limiting the required range of motion needed to execute a specific task. I refer to this stage as "clearing the runway." The remodeling phase requires a very specific type of manual work performed by a skilled body worker. To properly remodel soft tissue, the appropriate amount of *tension* must be placed in the affected areas to realign the soft tissue fibers. Tension is the key word and is very different from compression. My mentor Lenny used to say to me, "Tension works, compression hurts." Compression is a force that primarily, if not exclusively, goes directly into the tissue at a perpendicular angle. Tension is a tangential force which is applied more at a side angle. (Fig. 31). Both techniques have their purpose, but when trying to change the ability of a tissue to expand to its proper length, tension is what is necessary.

The great thing about the remodeling phase is that once you remodel something properly, you shouldn't need to do it over and over again. It would be analogous to cutting down trees in a forest to create a path. Once you knock down the trees, you don't come back the next day and cut the trees down again. That being said, if you don't use the path or maintain the path you created, brush and other growth can accumulate on the path. Soft tissues work the same way. Once you remodel and create a new pathway in the tissues, it is important to integrate that tissue into proper and efficient movements. This is the primary objective of the reprogramming phase.

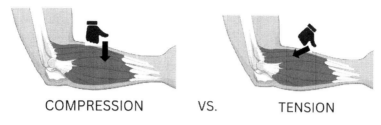

COMPRESSION   VS.   TENSION

Fig 31: Compression vs. Tension

The second best option, if a skilled body worker is not available, is to do some self-massage techniques using foam rollers and different body rolling balls. These are techniques that allow you to target specific areas, helping to optimize access to whatever your soft tissues have the capacity to give you without stronger intervention. All the exercises listed in the remodeling part of the Power Region Program use these types of modalities. The other thing that can be useful is getting a traditional deep tissue massage from a massage therapist. This tends to be more of a compressive approach, but a good deep tissue therapist can facilitate some new range of motion that can be helpful.

PHASE II: Reprogram

The reprogramming phase is an essential next step because you need to teach the body how to use and integrate the new motion that was created in the remodeling phase. When you create motion in an area that wasn't previously there, you've created naïve range of motion. It is very common for people to get off my table, after a soft tissue remodeling session, and feel a little wobbly. This is the body acclimating to the new range of motion. One thing I always do after remodeling an area is to have the client get off the table and immediately walk around. This allows the nervous system to integrate the new range of motion into the system ASAP, which is the initial part of reprogramming. The goal of the reprogramming phase is to integrate the new range of motion into a specific region, and then eventually integrate that successful reprogramming of the region into the foundational movement patterns. You can see examples of this in the Power Region Program, starting with a more isolated approach using foam rollers and balls to address specific muscles (rolling the bottom of the foot on a ball), and then progressing by integrating that muscle through a region specific motion (foot and ankle mobilization)—all based on the motion that this region needs to be able to do in order to perform the fundamental movement pattern, in this example, walking.

PHASE III: Conditioning

The conditioning phase is a continuation of reprogramming but increases the demand by challenging the region specific motion to build strength and endurance. These movements begin looking a little more like fundamental movement patterns of walking, lunging, and reaching and are designed to build resiliency and sustainability of proper movement. This phase ensures that the remodeling and reprogramming that has been done is sustainable over time and has resiliency to endure more loads and stresses.

PHASE IV: Enhance

The enhancement phase takes things to another level and includes movements that challenge the system a little more by going beyond one basic fundamental movement pattern.

This could look differently depending on the goal. The movements are usually much more dynamic and complex and require higher levels of coordination. In some cases unstable environments are introduced. An example of this is something I would do with my basketball and volleyball players to help them recover from and prevent ankle sprains. After properly progressing them through the basics, I introduce an unstable surface called an Airex pad where I have them perform the 3D Balance Foot Reach while passing a ball back and forth. I slowly increase the height of the passes until the arms of the athlete are completely above their head, to simulate what would happen in their sport.

CASE STUDY

"What are you going to do for me that ten other people haven't already done?"

My clinic in Southern California was commonly referred to as "The Last Resort." I frequently had individuals referred to me when they ran out of all other options. People showed up for their initial appointment and often told me that their friend said that they had to go to see "this guy" and that he might be able to help. I was "this guy."

In this particular situation, that was definitely the case. I had a gentleman come to see me whom I knew from the moment he walked in he didn't want to be there. His wife had pretty much dragged him in. He was in his late thirties and this poor guy had been to over ten different clinicians, therapists, doctors, and practitioners for his back pain. He was at the point where the only option left was a back surgery that they had told him might or might not help.

He sat in my office with his arms folded, looked me dead in the eye and asked, "What are you going to do with me that ten other people haven't already done?" I felt his frustration from across the room. This gentleman had already spent thousands and thousands of dollars on practitioners who had told him they could help him, but didn't.

I told him I didn't know if I could help him and that the first step would be to do a movement evaluation to see if there was a glaring biomechanical Big Rock that would potentially correlate to his pain.

After taking him through my assessment, there was a consistent Big Rock that showed up during many of his movements and was then confirmed with a table assessment, where I conducted a series of non-weight bearing range of motion tests. I was actually quite surprised because the degree of restriction I found in his right hip was significant. This was the Big Rock. When one of the Power Regions, in this case the hips, is not able to move properly and therefore load properly, it puts a tremendous strain on the back. It is like the 500 horsepower engine (the hips) is off and is asking the 100 horsepower engine (lumbar spine) to pick up the slack. I was surprised that it hadn't been addressed by the many practitioners he had seen. I shared with him what I believed was happening and that I believed I could help him.

He very sarcastically said, "Yeah I know, it's my hips causing my back pain because they are out of alignment. I've been down this road. I've already been told that, it's been addressed, and it hasn't helped."

This surprised me because if this hip imbalance was identified and addressed, why was he still presenting with it? I asked him what types of things these practitioners did with him to correct these imbalances. It then became clear why he still had the problem.

Although a few of these practitioners were able to identify the cause of the back pain, they didn't have the proper strategies to correct the imbalance. They all used the cadaveric-anatomy based strategies to treat the imbalance. They prescribed exercises like isolated muscle stretches and strengthening exercises for his hips, like clams and bridges, and performed the traditional soft tissue work, adjustments, and other modalities to address the symptom.

Why this gentleman's back was still in this condition and why he was not getting any results now made perfect sense. I felt relatively confident I could help him, but that didn't make him any less skeptical.

I realized anything I said was going to go into the category of lip service and fall on deaf ears, so I decided I wouldn't *tell* him I could help him. Instead, I would *show* him.

I offered to work with him for free until he felt that what I was doing was helping him. Once he felt like the service was worth it, he could start paying me for the sessions.

After two sessions of addressing his hip imbalance using the movement paradigm and principles, he had a 50 percent reduction of symptoms—more than he had received in the months of treatments he tried previously—and he could do more with less pain.

On his third session, he walked into my office, pulled out his credit card, and threw it on my desk, and said, "I guess it's time you get paid."

Trilogy of Vitality Pillar I Movement Summary

> ➤ Make sure to incorporate full body movements into your workout programs and do not exclusively train individual body parts
>
> ➤ Strength and flexibility are only relative to a specific task - there is no such thing as a person being "flexible" or "strong"
>
> ➤ The best way to maintain healthy neck, low back and knees is to keep your Power Regions accessible and strong for foundational movement patterns like walking, lunging, and squatting

TRILOGY OF VITALITY

PILLAR II: SYSTEMIC

Chapter 5

WE HAVE MASTERED HITTING THE BULLSEYE ON THE WRONG TARGET

Getting the body to move more efficiently will absolutely prevent unnecessary wear and tear overall but it will not heal anything. Healing, recovery, and growth happen from the inside out; it's a systemic process.

One thing I always share with my clients when they come in for help with injury recovery is that I have no ability to heal them. What I can do is put their bodies in the best possible position for their system to do the healing. In the few back pain case studies from chapters 3 and 4, I didn't "heal" their back pain. I improved the efficiency of the force distribution throughout their bodies to remove the unnecessary forces that were getting caught in their spine, causing pain. Any inflammation that was in the spine wasn't magically gone. Once the force was removed, the system was able to repair whatever damage had been done. This was assuming that the system had the capacity to heal and repair itself. There are many variables that contribute to the body's ability to heal and recover. This is what this chapter is all about.

Below you will find the five key variables that contribute directly to your systemic health, listed in order of importance. All five of these variables are always contributing to the state of everyone's systemic health and vitality. I will talk about all of these in this chapter but will focus mostly on nutrition.

1. Sleep
2. Getting Outside
3. Nutrition
4. Mental-Emotional
5. Movement

Sleep, There is NO Substitute

I thought I knew sleep was important until I read Matthew Walker's book, "Why We Sleep". After reading this book, making sure I was getting the adequate hours of sleep on a daily basis was now a non-negotiable part of my routine . Anytime I am helping one of my clients to organize and prioritize their day, the first thing I invite them to schedule and prioritize is getting their 7-9 hours of sleep. There is nothing you can do that will have a greater impact on your systemic health than getting adequate sleep. On the flip side, if you are not getting adequate sleep, there is nothing you can do to make up for its lack. If I am working with a client and they are only getting 4-6 hours of sleep a night or less, this becomes the priority. No amount of healthy eating, supplementation, or meditation can do what sleep does. These variables can help or hinder sleep but they cannot make up for not getting enough.

There are two strategies that I suggest to clients who are consistently getting less than 6 hours of sleep a night. The first and easiest to execute is committing to getting into bed 30 minutes earlier. This doesn't mean you have to be asleep 30 minutes earlier, but you want to initiate the sleep process a little earlier. When falling asleep and staying asleep for 7-9 hours is difficult, the best thing to do is to commit to resting the body for 7-9 hours a night. This means resting without stimulation from reading or screens, and sleeping for whatever duration is possible. There are a tremendous number of resources out there to help people get better sleep. I would recommend adding what you will learn in this chapter as part of your approach. The other four variables that I mentioned that contribute to creating systemic vitality also have a strong influence on the body's ability to sleep.

Getting Outside

The second most important aspect to creating systemic vitality is getting outside as much as you can throughout your day. The benefits of sunlight exposure and breathing in healthy fresh air are plentiful. The list of benefits just from daily sunlight exposure include better sleep, Vitamin D production, improved immunity, mood and motivation, stimulation of thyroid function, and prevention of depression. And, like sleep, there is no substitute for natural sunlight. There are, however, different types of Red Light therapy that mimic some of the beneficial light frequencies of the sun that can be supplemented during the winter. American neuroscientist and host of the "Huberman Lab Podcast", Andrew Huberman, went as far as to say in his "Maximizing Productivity" #28 Podcast: *"Getting sunlight in your eyes first thing in the morning is absolutely vital to mental and physical health. It is perhaps the most important thing that any and all of us can and should do in order to promote metabolic well-being, promote the positive functioning of your hormone system, and get your mental health steering in the right direction."*

I have been implementing Andrew's suggestion myself and I also highly recommend it to my clients. I make sure to get outdoors within 30-60 minutes of waking, and spend 10-30 minutes without sunglasses to get indirect sunlight into the eyes. I start every morning by taking my dog Barkley for a walk and make an effort to keep my gaze up to the sky, making sure never to look directly at the sun. My clients and I have seen phenomenal results in mood improvement and sustained motivation throughout the day when consistently implementing this simple practice.

The other habit that I strongly recommend is getting outside at least two additional times throughout your day for at least 10-30 minutes. Not only does this compound the benefits of sunlight exposure but it also breaks up the sitting that we tend to do when stuck indoors. One of the biggest downsides of being indoors all day is breathing in, indoor air. According to the EPA, indoor air quality can be 2-5x worse than outdoor air quality, even in industrialized cities[17]. The health problems linked to poor air quality include heart and lung disease, heart attacks, asthma, and other respiratory malfunctions. Getting some fresh air is critical to systemic health. There are even some plants you can keep in your home and office that help cleanse the air of pollutants. I have created a document that lists the best plants for air purity as well as air purifiers I recommend. Go to www.healthtovitality.com/resources.

While getting outside and getting fresh air is beneficial, you will optimize the time outside when you are breathing properly. Breathing is an action that we all do every day and most of us do not know how to do properly. In James Nestor's incredible book, "Breath, The New Science of a Lost Art", he shares what he has found to be the perfect breath.

---

[17] https://www.epa.gov/indoor-air-quality-iaq/inside-story-guide-indoor-air-quality

"Perfect breath" meaning optimizing the delivery of oxygen to the cells, stretching our lungs and straightening our bodies, improving blood flow, and absorbing all the benefits breathing offers us. He states that the perfect breath is an inhale for 5.5 seconds and an exhale of 5.5 seconds. I fulfill this cadence by simply doing a 6 second inhale and 6 second exhale. I start my day with this breath, focus on this cadence when I am walking outside, and when I am drifting off to sleep at night. I also intermittently practice it throughout my day when I remember or when taking a break in between clients or writing. This not only is systemically beneficial, but it is also psychologically beneficial. It reminds me to slow down and be more present.

Nutrition, Mental–Emotional, and Movement

The last three components that influence our systemic health are what we ingest, our mental-emotional state and how much we move or do not move. The Trilogy of Vitality addresses each of these three in great detail. In Chapters 3 and 4 I discussed the importance of movement and how to take care of the physical body. I will be taking a deep dive into the mental and emotional components in Chapters 7 and 8, so for the rest of this chapter, we are going to focus on nutrition.

I'm about to talk about Nutrition: Proceed with Caution

I have officially put the topic of nutrition in the same category as politics and religion. When I discuss nutrition, it's very much akin to discussing my beliefs about abortion, god, and immigration. Having conversations about any of these topics almost guarantees some fireworks. All three elicit strong emotions based on belief structures that many individuals are not willing to have open-minded discussions about. I have no intention of trying to convince you that my beliefs about nutrition are the right ones. There are many different ways to address nutrition and determine what we should be eating and what we shouldn't be eating. Points of contention don't even all have to do directly with food itself. Variables like animal cruelty, factory farming, global warming, carbon imprint, and countless other items are often part of this discussion.

That being said, the Vitality Principles of Eating that I will be sharing with you are based solely on what I have found to be the most supportive for myself, my family, and my clients to optimize and support our systemic bodies. It is most heavily biased on supporting Vitality. The evidence for this support is reflected in what I call the Vitality Big 6. As far as the scientific data and evidence of what I am going to share with you, I am heavily biased towards the scientific research of our nutrition mentor, Dr. Ray Peat. He is an independent scientist and his studies have not been and are not subsidized by any institutions, laboratories, or businesses. His guidance and recommendations have always produced exceptional results for myself, my family, and my clients - some of which I will be sharing with you. I will also be referencing many of Dr. Peat's articles throughout this chapter. You can find all his articles at www.raypeat.com.

My intention is to provide you with a perspective that I believe is very important and is definitely not readily available to the general public. I will warn you that a lot of what you are about to read will be very different from what you have been told by the mainstream media. I have strong beliefs about it, mostly because of the results I've seen them create. Ok, that's my disclaimer, if you have the *stomach* for it, let's dive into the Vitality Principles of Eating.

We are Hitting the Bullseye on the Wrong Target

When I think about nutrition or what foods are best for us to consume, I start by asking, "what's the goal?" The most fundamental goal of eating is to provide the fuel and the resources to enable the body to function at an optimal level. To put it simply, food is fuel and the materials for our bodies' to use to repair, recover, and grow. This is very different from getting people to lose weight (diet and exercise model) and keeping people alive (USDA recommendations). The objective behind the Vitality Principles of eating is to provide the body with the most optimal sources of fuel and raw materials to enable it to perform at its highest level possible. Unfortunately, when people come to me for nutritional support, that's not what they are asking for; and this is where the problem begins.

Two of the top reasons people come to me for an eating plan is to lose weight or to meet some "health marker" on their blood work, and a lot of times it is both. They are looking for a diet that will get the numbers on their blood work or the scale to change. Not only do they measure success by these two numbers, but somehow their health is also being measured by them. Keeping certain numbers in healthy ranges very rarely translates to a life of vitality.

I find that when people are focused on achieving the traditional "healthy numbers" using traditional protocols (whether it is weight, cholesterol, A1C, blood pressure, etc.) several other indicators are completely disregarded as not important enough to monitor. Neither are they recognized as indications that the "number" strategy is creating a lot of collateral damage and actually may be damaging our health. Targeting these arbitrary numbers as the mark to hit for health is focusing on hitting the bullseye on the wrong target. The indicators that are disregarded as being less important is what I believe need to be the primary focus. They are what I call the Vitality Big 6.

When our primary focus is on supplying our bodies with optimal fuel and raw materials, the body is able to function at an optimal level, the level of vitality. The Vitality Markers help us measure our vitality and there are six of them.

The Vitality Big 6

1. Quality of Sleep
2. Emotional Stability
3. Mental Acuity
4. Digestion
5. Energy Levels
6. Satiety

When I look at these six markers, I truly believe they are what we all want on a daily basis. When these six things are on point, life is good. The things we want and have to do seem possible, and vitality is the result. If one or more of these six things are off, it has a significant impact on our day-to-day experience. If one night we don't get a good night of sleep or when one bad night of sleep turns into a few days or a week, everything in our life is impacted from performance to simply enjoying our day. If our digestion is off, we feel bloated, constipated, or have pains in our stomach, it is hard to focus and concentrate on anything else.

On the flip side, when these six markers are measuring at a high level, it is easy to roll with the punches and to enjoy each and every day. Having a clear and sharp mind with sustainable energy levels throughout the day positions a person to optimize their time and fulfill the tasks that are most important for them to get done that day. We give our clients a document they can use to track their Big 6 by marking their scores each day, in the morning and throughout the day. This gives them a concrete way to monitor these markers and gauge the strategy they are implementing to ensure it is moving the needle on the dial toward vitality. The feedback also helps them chart the impact of the changes they are making in their diets and lifestyle. When individuals start to implement the Vitality Principles for eating, within a few days they normally begin to see a change in one or more of the six markers.

The other metric we use as a vitality indicator is resting body temperature. Body temperature is a great tool to monitor vitality in the body. If you have a healthy metabolism and are generating the proper amount of energy (heat), then your body should be running at about 98.2 degrees when first waking and about 98.6 degrees in the middle of the day.[18] If you would like a copy of the form below so you are able to track your Vitality Big 6 and temperatures, go to www. healthtovitality.com/resources

---

[18] Peat Ray (2007)

Wake Up Time	Resting Body Temperature Morning	Resting Body Temperature Mid-Afternoon	Quality of Sleep 1-terrible 10-amazing	Bedtime

Time	Satiety 1-Not Hungry 10- Starving	Energy 1-Sluggish 10-Hyper	Emotions 1-depressed 2-irritable	Focus 1-Foggy 10-Scattered	Digestion (G)Gas, (B)urps, (C)onstipated, (D)iarrhea

Time to Aim for a Different Target

Countless clients have come to me over the years who had "healthy blood work", but were experiencing sleep problems, mood swings, energy crashes, and all kinds of digestive issues. Now let me be clear, I am not saying blood work doesn't have a place and doesn't provide us with valuable information. I am saying we need to keep things in perspective. Blood work tells part of the story, and it is a snapshot of what is happening. Over the years, the amount of extrapolation I have seen made from one blood test has been astonishing. To think we know the whole story from one test would be like looking at a single freeze frame of a movie and thinking we know the entire movie plot. I have had cases where people came in because overall, they just felt unwell. They reported having symptoms like fatigue, being overweight, having trouble focusing, and experiencing aches and pains. But their blood work said everything looked good, just like my elbow X-ray.

I've also had the flip side happen. A client feels good, has high energy and is active, yet their blood work indicates they are not healthy because their cholesterol or A1C is too high. They are then put on medications to get their blood work to look better. Suddenly their energy level goes down and they have body aches.

One class of medications I have found to cause the most problems for people are statin drugs. One gentleman came to me for help with his nutrition because he was prescribed statins for "high cholesterol". Prior to his diagnosis, he was a super active, high energy leader of a large construction firm, and very fit. Once on the statins, he developed all kinds of muscle and body aches, suffering from fatigue and low energy. He took himself off them within the first month..

One thing I always make an effort to do in these cases is to educate my clients on what cholesterol *actually* is, since it has been wrongly vilified by the "health" model. Turns out, cholesterol is not this evil villain that your body produces to create heart attacks. Cholesterol is the precursor to every steroid and sex hormone your body makes. Without cholesterol there is no testosterone, DHEA, estrogen, progesterone, or pregnenolone which are all essential hormones that the body needs for optimal function. Vitamin D is also a byproduct of the synthesis of cholesterol.

When someone has "high levels of cholesterol", instead of artificially restricting the body from producing it, what we should be asking is why isn't the cholesterol being converted over to these essential resources? Interestingly enough, hypothyroidism used to be diagnosed by high levels of cholesterol because thyroid hormone and Vitamin A must be present for cholesterol to be converted over into these essential products. So if there are high levels of cholesterol measured in the blood, it was thought that there wasn't enough thyroid hormone being produced, specifically Triiodothyronine (also known as T_3), to convert the cholesterol over. In Dr. Ray Peat's article, "Cholesterol, Longevity, Intelligence, and Health", he shares the other side of the cholesterol story that I believe everyone should read.

The best results I have seen for individuals, including myself, is to incorporate *all* the information from tests like bloodwork with your Vitality Markers and weigh the Vitality Markers a little heavier than any specific test. If the Vitality Markers are all at healthy levels, there is a good chance the system is operating at a high level, even if some numbers may be "off" according to some arbitrary data of "healthy" ranges that happen to be directly correlated to the "need" to take medication.

The reality we must all face, is that when certain tests are linked to qualifying a patient for a specific prescription medication, there are *billions* of dollars on the line—this is not a small variable. Cholesterol is a perfect example of this. When you get a lipoprotein panel included in your blood work, which is pretty standard, you will get a measure of the total cholesterol found in your blood. Today if you measure around 200 mg/dl of cholesterol in your blood, you are placed in the category of "high cholesterol" and are eligible for statins. In the 1980s, high cholesterol was considered to be 240 mg/dl or higher[19] and in the 1990s, the marker for high cholesterol was 20 points lower at 220 mg/dl.[20] Every time this number drops, the market for statin drugs exponentially grows. The market value of statin drugs in 2021 was just under 15 billion dollars and is projected to be over 20 billion dollars by 2029.[21] Does this mean these companies don't care about people and aren't trying to help them? I'd like to believe that isn't the case, but the facts are the facts.

The Vitality Principles for Eating

When it comes to recommendations on nutrition, I do not believe there is a one-size-fits-all way of eating. There are many variables that influence what foods are best for each and every individual at a given time in their life. Some of those variables include ethnicity, age, and current level of health. I will say, however, that following the Vitality Principles for Eating have consistently supported individuals

---

[19] Burke Gregory et al. (1991)
[20] Schucker B et al. (1991)
[21] Alliance News Via Comtex (2022)

in experiencing greater vitality in their lives. And as I stated earlier, the way I define "greater vitality" is an improvement in the Vitality Big 6 and resting body temperature. Most of the evidence I have for this is clinical and from the results Eve and I have seen with clients.

I'd like to share a few recent cases that Eve and I have had. We used the Vitality Principles for Eating to support individuals with a variety of issues. Implementing these principles helped several people who had severe digestive issues, most recently chronic diarrhea. This was cleared up in a few weeks. We also worked with a young woman who wanted to conceive and had been told it would be very difficult because she was too overweight and her hormones were out of balance. We helped her to optimize her Vitality Big 6 and within a year, she not only had lost weight but was able to conceive her first child. Two other clients struggled daily with chronic fatigue and had chronic urinary tract infections; both were eliminated within a few months of implementing these principles. Other ailments that we have seen significantly improve, and in many cases, completely eliminated, include insomnia, headaches, constipation, brain fog, and emotional instability. In some of these cases, Eve has also integrated homeopathic protocols but all of them started with the Vitality Principles of Eating.

I am going to present to you what I have found for myself and for others to consistently deliver the greatest global impact on the systemic health of the body. Below is the general macronutrient breakdown as well as the ideal types of macronutrients

The Vitality Paradigm
Macronutrient Breakdown

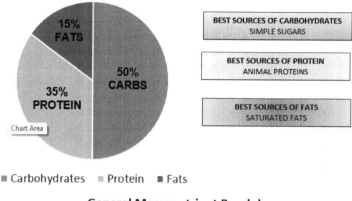

Carbohydrates   Protein   Fats

General Macronutrient Breakdown

Fats ≤ Protein ≤ Carbohydrates

These recommendations are focused on the things that put the body in an optimal environment to operate at its highest level. The Vitality Principles for systemic health are all things that support your body to make cellular energy, recover, repair, grow and develop. These are the basic functions that are needed for everything else in the system to work. When these basic needs are not addressed, there is a cascade of symptoms that manifest which negatively impact the vitality markers: terrible sleep, energy crashes, mood swings, digestive issues, brain fog, and cravings. The above graphic gives you the general idea. Now, let's break down the details on the different macronutrient recommendations. First stop, carbohydrates.

Sugar is Your Friend

If there is one macronutrient that needs to hire a better PR (Public Relations) Firm, it's sugar. Sugar gets blamed for everything these days. I often hear people say they are cutting out sugars in an attempt to be healthier. I always ask them what they mean by sugar and often get responses like, "I've cut back on cookies, crackers, cakes, and other desserts." Or they will say, "muffins, bagels, pastas, cereals and breads." The thing that makes these foods unhealthy is not the sugar they contain. You'd be fortunate if there were any real sugar in these foods. Many of them are made with artificial sweeteners like high fructose corn syrup as well as other additives. The most harmful ingredients in these foods are the flour and grains - not the sugar! It has gotten so bad that now I even hear people say they don't eat fruit or honey because it has sugar!?! This has officially gotten out of control. I would say sugar gets blamed for what flour, processed oils, and artificial sweeteners are doing to our health. Sugar is **not** the problem.[22]

Sugar is a carbohydrate and more specifically a substance called sucrose. Sucrose is a disaccharide made up of glucose and fructose. I will be talking about the significance of this combination later in this section. Carbohydrates are our primary source of glucose. Glucose is an essential source of energy in all organisms. It gives every cell in your body energy. Without glucose, your body would break down and die. Insulin is the chemical that carries the glucose into the cell for fuel. When these systems are working optimally, they

---

[22] And for those of you saying, *"What about cancer Matt?!? Sugar is the worst thing for cancer?!",* I'd recommend entertaining a different perspective and refer you to two of Dr. Peat's articles, "Cancer: Disorder and Energy" and "The Caner Matrix."

maintain healthy blood sugar levels which are essential for survival. Many of us have experienced the effects of low blood sugar. Symptoms of low blood sugar include increased heart rate, sweating, nervousness, anxiety, dizziness, and irritation. I will be sharing with you why, eating naturally occurring simple sugars, root vegetables, and tubers as your primary source of carbohydrates gets glucose to the cell for oxidative metabolism in the most efficient - and natural - way.

The carbohydrates that seem to create the most problems when eaten in high volumes are the grains, beans, legumes, pastas, and rice. Yes, the very thing we are told by the USDA to eat most of. I call these carbohydrate sources the survival foods. They are by far the cheapest to produce and will ensure survival when eaten at high volumes, but they create a plethora of side effects. The most common side effects when you eat high volumes of these foods are digestive issues. Beans and legumes create such a consistent digestive problem that we created a catchy song about it: "Beans, beans, the musical fruit, the more you eat, the more you toot." Now although some gas is normal, beans take things to a whole other level. Beans frequently cause flatulence, stomach pain, and bloating because they contain a fiber called raffinose that causes digestive problems.[23] And we have already talked about grains producing digestive issues. A common solution is to find ways to prepare beans and grains to modify them to minimize the side effects, like soaking the beans and grains before cooking and ingesting them. This just doesn't make sense to me. If we have to go through this much trouble to make sure these foods don't hurt us, maybe we should consider that these foods aren't ideal for us to eat.

I've referred to two types of carbohydrates, simple sugars and complex carbohydrates. Let's explore their different

---

[23] Link Rachael (2021)

characteristics further. Simple carbohydrates, like those found in fruits, are broken down and converted to energy quickly. Complex carbohydrates take longer to digest and break down more slowly due to their molecular structure. The other significant difference between simple and complex carbohydrates is that simple sugars contain sucrose while the complex sugars contain glucose. Remember that sucrose is made up of two saccharides; glucose and fructose. The reason this is significant is because the combination of these two saccharides equate to a more consistent blood sugar level. If we look at the glycemic index,[24] it tells us that glucose has a value of 100, fructose is the lowest at 23 and sucrose is 65 (Fig 32). The combination of the high value of glucose and the low value of fructose equals a strong but sustainable value when combined. This is why simple sugars (sucrose)are favorable.

	Glycemic Index Value
Glucose	100
Sucrose	65
Fructose	23

Fig 32: Glycemic Values of glucose, sucrose, and fructose

The fact that it takes more time for complex carbohydrates to be broken down creates an illusion that it is better for maintaining blood sugar levels, especially when you look at glycemic index values like black beans sitting at a value of 33, compared to an orange that sits at a value of 40. The thing that isn't well known, and therefore not taken into consideration, is that the glycemic index of foods is a measure of sugar in the bloodstream two hours after ingestion. When

---

[24] The University of Sydney (2022)

you measure blood sugar levels of black beans an hour later, it rises 52% to a value of 50. An orange increases by only 20% to a value of 48. We want a steady flow of glucose, not a large spike, making an orange much more favorable.

Dr. Ray Peat, in his article "Glycemia, Starch, and Sugar in Context" explains how misleading the glycemic index is and how it unfairly paints simple carbohydrates as the problem and complex carbohydrates as the solution.[25] As Dr. Peat shares in his article, one of the main reasons why simple sugars (sucrose) sustain blood sugar more efficiently than complex carbohydrates, is the role fructose plays in inhibiting the stimulation of insulin from glucose. This levels out the delivery of glucose into the cells. Simple sugars like fruits also have a variety of other benefits as a primary source of carbohydrates. One being, the concentration of essential vitamins and minerals. Some vitamins and minerals, like potassium, also help regulate blood sugar levels. He even goes as far as to say:

> *"Eating complex carbohydrates, rather than sugars, is a reasonable way to promote obesity. Eating starch, by increasing insulin and lowering the blood sugar, stimulates the appetite, causing a person to eat more, so the effect on fat production becomes much larger than when equal amounts of sugar and starch are eaten."*

If we want sustainable levels of blood sugar, then simple sugars are the better choice.

The other factor that is important to consider when looking at some of the "healthy" complex carbohydrate recommendations are the other characteristics that these

---

[25] Peat Ray (2009)

types of carbohydrates tend to have. I have found that many of the recommended "healthy" complex carbohydrates create a myriad of side effects for people. The ones I would be most mindful of are beans, seeds and legumes. We have found that eliminating these three foods from a client's diet has created the greatest impact in overall vitality then any other modification. Beans, seeds, and legumes, universally, have created the most amount of digestive and blood sugar issues for the clients Eve and I have worked with over the last twenty years.

The absolute best source of carbohydrates to maintain blood sugar and optimize glucose delivery to the cells are fruits and dairy. The best complex carbohydrates are tubers. The reason why tubers are the best vegetables is because they are grown below the ground. Being below the ground means they are more protected from being eaten by animals. This is significant because they therefore do not contain harmful substances that are meant to be deterrents to being eaten. This makes them more friendly to our digestive system. In addition, tubers are also known as the storage organs for nutrients in some plants - giving them numerous nutritional benefits. In the next chapter, you will see a chart with 4 Food Groups. Group I foods are the best food sources and include a list of these optimal fruits and vegetables.

While getting fuel to the cells is essential to the body's ability to function optimally, we must also make sure to provide the body with the necessary raw materials to repair and regenerate itself. This is where protein comes in.

Solidifying Your Infrastructure

When I think of protein, I think of raw materials that are needed to build something. If I was going to build a home, I would need to gather concrete, wood, rebar, braces, nails, screws, and a variety of other materials. Without these things, there would be no house. It is also important to note that when something needs repair in your house, you need new raw materials to repair what is worn or broken. Protein plays this exact role in our bodies. Without protein, there is no repairing anything in the body. Protein provides the infrastructure and resources for all the systems and processes of the body.

A common situation I run into when working with a client who has come to me to physically rehabilitate an injury, is that they are not eating enough of the right kinds of protein. This makes healing more challenging. It is critical to supply the body with ample amounts of protein when looking to recover and repair the body from injury. It is the protein that repairs and heals what's broken. In this section I will share with you the optimal protein sources to repair and regenerate all systems of the body. Before we go there, let's talk about what proteins are made of.

Proteins are made up of chains of amino acids. There are a total of twenty-seven amino acids, each having unique functions in the body. These amino acids are the building blocks for everything in the body, including muscle, connective tissue, hormones, enzymes, neurotransmitters, skin, nails, and hair, to name a few. Different protein sources contain different amino acid profiles. What this means is that not all amino acids are in all protein sources. In addition different amino acids are designed to do different things. You can think of amino acids as different types of raw materials. Like the house analogy, some amino acid profiles act like "wood and screws", while others function as "electrical wire and brackets." Each is used for something different in the house.

In general, there are two protein sources—animal and vegetable. Animal proteins are complete and contain all of the amino acids we need for repair and healing; these include dairy, eggs, meats, and bone broths. The combination of these sources provide the full spectrum of amino acids needed by the body. The only foods I relate to as sources of protein are the animal protein sources, even though there is protein in other sources.

Vegetable protein is not a complete protein source and require a much higher volume and a higher degree of supplementation to get all the amino acids our bodies' need. Sources like soy, tofu, legumes, beans, nuts, and seeds also contain many substances that are not supportive of and in some cases inhibitive to optimal metabolic function. In addition to these poor sources of protein, many of the vegan and vegetarian options that are available contain chemicals like dipotassium phosphate, potassium chloride, titanium dioxide and maltodextrin to name a few. All of which have been shown to have a myriad of harmful side effects.[26] If it takes this much work and tinkering to get vegetables to taste and do the job of meat, maybe we should just be eating meat?

Is it possible to get all the necessary amino acids as a vegetarian while minimizing the side effects of these foods? I guess it's possible, but it takes a tremendous amount of effort and supplementation if you were ever going to pull it off. I don'tI know many people who can pull it off in a healthy way, not to mention in a way that leads to vitality. The amount of preparation, meticulous calculation, and combinations of foods, coupled with the volume and supplementation necessary to get it done properly, equates to what I'd consider to be a part-time job. For this reason, I do not see it as the ideal way to meet the body's protein needs. Again, because of the massive effort needed to pull it off, one could conclude

---

[26] https://www.consumerfreedom.com/2021/07/5-chemicals-lurking-in-plant-based-meats/

that the body wasn't really designed to be vegan or vegetarian. Not to mention that animals that are vegetarian, herbivores, have completely different digestive systems than humans. Their digestive systems are designed to breakdown grasses and other vegetation. Humans, who are omnivores, have completely different digestive systems.

Let me just say, I am aware that some of you are reacting like you just found out my views on abortion are different than yours and may be reading this and getting upset. Some may disregard this chapter, skip it, or even dismiss everything else in this book. That is certainly your right and your choice. But, before you do that, if you were feeling compelled to do so, I do want you to know that I completely respect and totally understand anyone who is vegetarian because of the cruelty to animals and the impact factory farming has on our environment. I have good friends who are vegetarian and vegan who feel this way, and I support them completely.

However, most, if not all of them, struggle with their health and more specifically the Vitality Markers. A few of them, when their health was bad enough, started integrating animal protein sources into their diets and many of their health issues began to diminish. If you are someone who has figured out how to integrate vegetarianism into your lifestyle and score high on the vitality markers, then well done. I haven't seen this to be an easy feat, and if you are vegan or vegetarian and are struggling with your health and most importantly the Vitality Markers, I would consider integrating some animal protein sources into your routine. There are incredible resources for finding farms that are raising animals humanely and sustainably. Below are some resources that provide sources and perspectives on sustainable and humane farming, while maintaining a state of reverence for the animals.

Must see documentaries: *Food Inc.*, *Chef's Table* Vol. 6, Ep. 2

Sources for humane farming: eatwild.com, grasslandbeef. com, westonaprice.org

---

The final thing to note about protein is that profiles of different amino acids serve different purposes. Some amino acids are geared toward growth and development and others are geared toward recovery and regeneration. Foods falling into the category of growth and development are therefore more stimulating to the system, including foods like muscle meats, whey protein, egg whites, and milk. Muscle meats are essentially any piece of meat, steak, chicken, pork, or ground beef. Foods that have more of the regenerative amino acid profile include homemade bone broths, cheese, gelatin supplements, and yolks.

Amino acids found in the connective tissue of animals, like bones, ligaments, and skin, contain higher amounts of amino acids like glycine, proline, hydroxyproline, and lysine which perform more of the maintenance and repair functions of the body. The proper ratios of how much of each of these two types of proteins is ideal to eat, vary based on your age., The further you are away from puberty, the less growth and development is necessary. Therefore the proteins designed for growth and development (like muscle meats) are not as necessary. A good general rule of thumb is to aim for a 60:40 ratio of muscle meats to connective tissue up to puberty. As you age, slowly progressing the ratio to a 20:80 ratio up into your later years in life. You can read more about this in Dr. Peats article, "Gelatin, stress, longevity".

Now that you know how to use carbohydrates and protein to provide the ideal fuel and resources for growth, repair, and recovery, it's time to discuss fats. What you will discover in the next section is that some of the fats you are currently eating could be the most damaging thing you are consuming when it comes to your vitality. And it is not the fats you think.

Avoid Poly

Fats have always been a hot topic when it comes to nutrition. The recommendations on what fats are good and what fats are bad are always changing. At one time, saturated fats were poison and you were told you should be eating margarine and shortening. Then it was discovered that trans fats were really the enemy. Now with Paleo and Keto diets all the rage, people are eating a tremendous amount of fat, "to be healthy". Once again, the basis for many of these recommendations continues to overlook the most basic biological needs of our bodies and over complicate everything. I am going to break down some of the most basic facts about the two types of fats, saturated and unsaturated fats, and specifically focus on polyunsaturated fats. I hope this creates clarity on what we should really be avoiding.

Let's start by defining the two fats, saturated and unsaturated. Unsaturated fats are fatty acid molecules that contain one or more double bonds in their chemical structure. Saturated fats are fatty acids that have no double bonds. The greater the degree of unsaturation (the more double bonds) the more susceptible the fatty acid is to turning rancid. Rancidity is called *lipid peroxidation*. It happens when an oxygen molecule binds to one of the extra bonds, causing an oxidation of the molecule. This oxidized molecule is called a free radical. Free radicals are known to adversely alter lipids, protein, and DNA leading to a number of human diseases, including diabetes, heart disease and cancer.[27] To put it simply, we don't want to consume high volumes of foods that go rancid and create free radicals in the body.

A _poly_unsaturated fat means it is *very* unsaturated or it has *many* double bonds which could also be translated as being *very* unstable and highly likely to oxidize. Not only does the binding of oxygen create high levels of free radicals but it robs the body of oxygen that could be put to better use. Oxygen in the body means energy in the body. When Eve and I cut out the foods high in polyunsaturated oils we saw an immediate increase of energy day in and day out.

There is one other type of fat to mention and that is a monounsaturated fat. Monounsaturated fats only have one double bond so they are more stable than polyunsaturated fats but not as stable as saturated fat. Olive oil is an example of a great monounsaturated fat when used as a garnish or for cooking at low heat. The smoke point when using olive oil for cooking should be somewhere around 370-405⁰ F. Higher heats can cause it to go rancid, like the polyunsaturated fats.

I firmly believe the most dangerous foods that the American population consumes on a daily basis are foods that have high amounts of polyunsaturated fats. Dr. Ray Peat has done extensive research on this topic of fats and it is summarized well in his article, *"Suitable Fats, Unsuitable Fats: Issues in Nutrition"*[28]. Clinically, I have found that clients who have done *nothing* else but limited or eliminated food high in polyunsaturated fats have seen the greatest impact in their vitality—more than from any other simple change.

I also want to address the ideas of "essential fatty acids" and the "importance of omega-3 fatty acids". I believe that

---

[27] Dix Megan (2018)
[28] Peat Ray (2007)

these ideas are significantly overstressed and the fact that there is a billion dollar industry attached to these supplements just amplifies my skepticism. Most, if not all the studies that speak to the importance of these fats, are directly correlated to this billion dollar industry. I am not saying that omega 3, 6, and 9 fatty acids aren't important and don't play a critical role in our vitality, but it is definitely not something we need to be supplementing with or focused on to the extent that we are. Eating the proper sources of the vitality foods will provide more than enough of these substances. If anything, I have had more success decreasing the amount of these substances in my diet and in the diets of my clients. Dr. Peat has some excellent articles on this very subject but the two I'd recommend reading are, "Unsaturated Fatty Acids: Nutritionally Essential, or Toxic?" and "The Great Fish Oil Experiment". Let's talk about the fats that I believe are truly essential to vitality.

Saturated fats are much more stable fats because they do not have those double chemical bonds. This makes their molecular structure more tolerant of heat and oxygen, which our body is filled with, ensuring that they do not become rancid when ingested. These fats are usually in solid form at room temperature, like butter, coconut oil, tallow and lard.

Fats like flaxseed oil, canola oil, soybean oil, and vegetable oil are all liquid at room temperature. You may have even noticed that when you see flaxseed oil sold in the store, it is usually in a dark container and refrigerated. This is to protect it so it doesn't get exposed to light or heat and go rancid. You may have also noticed when you take off the cap of the flaxseed, canola, and vegetable oil containers, it tends to be sticky. That is oxidized oil that has gone rancid. Can you imagine what that looks like in the body after you ingest it? Picture that stickiness clogging up your arterial walls. These are the oils that you want to avoid like the plague!

Unfortunately, when you read the label on most packaged foods, you will see at least one of these types of oils listed as one of the main ingredients.

Now, for those of you who might be thinking, *"what about saturated fats and their role in high cholesterol and heart attacks?"* The myth of the correlation between saturated fats and cholesterol as the primary cause of heart problems has been slowly deteriorating over the last twenty years. Without going down too much of a rabbit hole with this topic, I will refer you to Dr. Peat's article "Cholesterol, Longevity, Intelligence, and Health" and remind you about the role cholesterol actually plays. I'll also share an interesting fact that studies have shown that 70 percent of the plaques blocking arteries are <u>un</u>saturated fats.[29]

This is a topic that can take up an entire book and I am not the person to write that book but I can definitely share some excellent ones that have been written on this subject. A few of my favorites include:

- *Saturated Fat May Save Your Life* by Bruce Fife
- *The Great Cholesterol Con* by Anthony Colpo
- The Great Cholesterol Myth, Revised and Expanded" by Dr. John Bowden

Another Reason to Avoid Beans and Legumes

Previously I mentioned that beans and legumes are not the greatest sources of protein because they are incomplete in their amino acid profile and have fibers in them that create digestive issues. There is an additional downside to beans and legumes. They have high levels of polyunsaturated fats. For

[29] Felton C et al. (1997)

all of these reasons, you will find beans and legumes on the list of foods to limit or avoid.

Below is a list of oils that you will find in many foods, especially processed foods, that contain the highest percentage of polyunsaturated fats (Fig 33). If Eve and I see any of these oils in the ingredients of anything we pick up in the grocery store, we immediately place it back on the shelf; I'd recommend that you do the same thing.

OILS HIGH IN POLYUNSATURATED FATS	
Safflower Oil	78%
Sunflower Oil	69%
Walnut Oil	66%
Corn Oil	62%
Soybean Oil	61%
Cottonseed Oil	54%
Sesame Oil	43%
Peanut Oil	34%
Canola Oil	31%
Apricot Oil	31%

Fig 33: Percentage of polyunsaturated fats in oils

CASE STUDY

"Eve's Story"

Eve was a vegetarian—primarily because of the cruelty inflicted on the animals raised for meat. She ate a high volume of beans, rice, tofu, grains, greens, and other vegetables, and the occasional cheese or egg. Eve had been struggling with a myriad of systemic issues. The most chronic and painful were menstrual issues, ovarian cysts, and monthly urinary tract infections. Eve's case study is one of the strongest illustrations of the power of the Vitality Principles of Eating I can share with you. It was made even more powerful because I was involved in her journey on a day to day basis.

When we sought support from the traditional medical model, she was offered modifications to her birth control pills and given other types of medications that didn't help. At one point, she was told that getting pregnant would be very difficult. This was devastating news as she was in her mid-twenties and having children was something we planned and looked forward to. It got to the point where nothing was helping and she was presented with her next, and only, option—a hysterectomy.

Around this time, I was starting my deep dive into studying nutrition and systemic health. I was taking different courses, getting different certifications, and eventually signed up to be certified in a program called Metabolic Typing. The instructor was Dodie Anderson and she had been studying nutrition and working as a nutritionist for over 30 years when I met her. She had engaged and studied every diet that existed. She was a wealth of knowledge. After giving the level one certification, she asked for feedback on the course. I was happy to share my thoughts but wasn't sure how happy she was going to be with them. I told her that there was phenomenal information in the course, things I'd never heard anywhere else. However, I thought the whole metabolic typing testing and recommendations were just a money grab. It didn't seem to make sense to me or be helpful.

After I shared this, I was expecting her to hang up on me, but instead, after a brief period of silence, she said she agreed with everything I said. I asked her why she was teaching things if she didn't agree with them. She then explained that she had been studying with a nutritional scientist named Dr. Ray Peat and she was learning from him all of the information that I thought was so unique and powerful. Dodie then shared that she had been trying to incorporate this into the curriculum more and more.

After that conversation, I asked Dodie if I could come down to La Jolla, San Diego, every week from Los Angeles and study with her. I told her I wanted to know everything she was learning. So for the next year, Dodie took Eve and me under her wing, with the guidance of Dr. Ray Peat, and taught us some of the key concepts you will find inside of the Vitality Principles of Eating.

As we began learning from Dodie and Ray, we started to implement these new principles of eating in our own lives. One of the first things they had us do was to track Eve's Vitality Big 6 and to take her temperature in the morning and afternoon. It was no surprise that her Vitality Big 6 was not great. She wasn't sleeping very well, her energy levels were low, she felt bloated and frequently had stomach pains. She also had periods of time when it was hard for her to concentrate and was emotionally all over the map. Her morning temperature was no higher than 96.5 degrees and it never got above 97.2 degrees at any point during the day. All of this was a serious indication that her system and more specifically her metabolism was not operating at an optimal level.

We slowly eliminated all foods that were anti-metabolic and pro-inflammatory like beans, wheat, soy products, certain greens, and any food that contained polyunsaturated fats. This basically meant she needed to slowly eliminate everything she had been eating except the cheese and eggs. She began to change her diet, eating more fruits and becoming more open to eating some muscle meats and homemade bone broths. We learned about farmers who not only raised their livestock humanely but operated with a state of reverence and respect for the animals they were raising.

After implementing this new way of eating for a few months, her Vitality Big 6 symptoms began improving and her body temperatures began to slowly rise. She also went two months without a urinary tract infection, which was unheard of at that point. These were all very good signs and she was very encouraged.

But the major evidence that her diet had been responsible for her physical ailments came a few months later, when she went back to her OB/GYN for a progress report on her cysts. When I first saw her after her appointment, she walked into our bedroom with tears in her eyes. I immediately thought she had received terrible news - that things were not improving and that surgery was inevitable. To my surprise they were tears of joy—her doctor reported that there was no sign of cysts on her scan and all other tests looked good!!

I'll never forget that day. I remember we immediately began trying to conceive our first child because we thought it would take time after to conceive a child after all we had been through. Well, as it turned out, a few weeks later when I came home, Eve was standing in the hallway with a big smile on her face. I couldn't believe it—she was pregnant! About eight months later, she gave birth to a beautiful, healthy baby boy whom we named Christian. Christian is now fourteen years old and was joined six years later by his sister, Emma.

When I start introducing individuals to the Vitality Paradigm of eating, it is always fun seeing life come back into their eyes, because I know exactly what it feels like.

Chapter 6

THE VITALITY FOODS

Below is the Vitality Food Pyramid. (Fig 34) This will give you a general idea of what we consider to be the Vitality Foods. These foods provide the body with the optimal resources to make cellular energy and to repair and regenerate itself. In the following pages, I will give you examples of each part of the Vitality Food Pyramid and break down why the foods are in each of the categories.

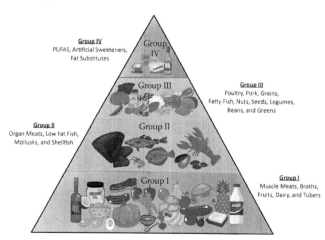

Fig 34: The Vitality Food Pyramid

Here is a further breakdown of each of the groups of foods.
(Fig 35)

GROUP 1 FOODS
These are the core foods of your diet and make up
the majority of what you are eating.

Muscle Meats	Homemade Broths	Vegetables	Fruits	
Beef	Beef	Potatoes	Apples	
Buffalo	Chicken	Carrots	Apricots	
Lamb		Pumpkin	Bananas	Papaya
Venison	**Fats**	Squash	Cherries	Peaches
	Butter	Yams	Grapefruit	Pears
Dairy	Coconut Oil	Cucumbers	Melons	Pineapple
Milk	Olive Oil	Peppers	Nectarines	Plums
Cheese	Ghee	Tomatoes	Oranges	Fresh Fruit Juices
Eggs	Tallow			

GROUP 2 FOODS
These foods supply large quantities of essential vitamins & minerals. These are
best to supplement into your diet 1-2x per week varying each week.

Organ Meats	Low Fat Fish	Shellfish	
Fresh Beef Liver	Flounder	Shrimp	
Fresh Wild Game Liver	Cod	Lobster	Clams
Heart	Sole	Mussels	Oysters
Kidney	Mahi Mahi		

GROUP 3 FOODS
These foods are ones to eat with caution. Eat Group 3 foods, no more than 1-3x a month.

Poultry & Pork		Grains	Fatty Fish	Vegetables
Chicken	Pheasant	Breads	Salmon	Broccoli
Turkey	Bacon	Pastas	Swordfish	Cauliflower
Duck	Ham	Rice	Tuna	Beans & Legumes
Pork Ribs		**Nuts & Seeds**	Halibut	Greens

GROUP 4 FOODS
AVOID as much as possible

OILS		Fat Substitutes	Trans Fats
Corn	Sesame	Carrageenan	Margarine
Soybean	Peanut	All the "gums"	Crisco
Safflower	Apricot		
Flaxseed	Cottonseed	**Artificial Sweeteners**	
Fish Oils	Canola	High Fructose Corn Syrup	
Sunflower	Walnut	Aspartame	
		Saccharin	**Soy Products & Hydrogenated Oils**
		Sucralose	

Group 1 Foods

Group 1 foods make up the majority of your preferred calories. Different combinations of these foods can be eaten on a daily basis. The only caveat to this are the muscle meats. Depending on your age (See "Solidifying Infrastructure" section in chapter 5) you may only be consuming muscle meats 1-2 times a week and having homemade broths and soups more frequently. Not only do Group 1 foods provide the body with the best sources of protein, fat, and carbohydrates, but they also do not contain high amounts of the anti-metabolic and anti-digestion substances found in Group 3 and Group 4 foods.

The reason you only see red meat in this section is because the digestive systems of herbivores animals like cows, bison, and sheep have digestive systems that have the ability to convert the unsaturated fats they consume into saturated fats. This ensures that when we eat red meats, we are consuming mostly saturated fats, regardless of the animal's diet. Poultry and swine, on the other hand, because they are not herbivores and have different digestive systems, are unable to convert the unsaturated fats, in their feed, into saturated fat. The only way around this is to find wild poultry and swine that do not have diets supplemented with grain products. In these cases, their diets do not have high amounts of unsaturated fats so are much better for humans to eat. This is also why I prefer tallow (from cattle) to lard (from pig).

This brings me to another very important topic, food quality. Food quality is one of the most important variables to consider when it comes to consuming anything, especially animal products. My dear friend and family doctor, Dr. Yoshi Rahm, said to me once, "Meat is one of the healthiest foods you can eat and meat can also be one of the most unhealthy foods you can eat." He was referring to the source and therefore the quality of the meat. For the resources on high quality animal products, refer back to chapter 5 where I discuss "Solidifying Your Infrastructure".

On the subject of dairy, it is important to mention that some individuals have some degree of dairy sensitivity. Eve and I have worked with individuals who are dairy sensitive and have had a lot of success slowly introducing these individuals to raw milk dairy products. We believe it is by far the healthiest form of dairy for our bodies. We and our children have been consuming raw milk and other raw milk dairy products for the last 15 years. It is one of the most nutrient dense and one of the last real authentic foods available to us. Since so many of our foods are processed, it's nice to have one thing that is natural. The intolerance to dairy may very well be a barometer of a person's digestive health. Healing the gut by eliminating the Group 4 foods and limiting the Group 3 foods, will generally allow individuals to tolerate dairy again. If you would like more information on dairy and raw milk, I would highly recommend reading "The Untold Story of Milk" by Ron Schmid.

I will also mention that I am not a proponent of alternative dairy substitutes like soy milk and almond milk. First and foremost, it isn't milk. I've never seen a soybean or an almond with breasts. When you add this to all the issues I have already raised with beans, legumes, nuts, and seeds, I believe it makes these "milk" sources more harmful than beneficial. All of that being said, we know there are exceptions to everything and we all must do what we feel is best for our own bodies.

NOTE: Two excellent resources to find high quality sources of raw dairy in your area are realmilk.com and westonaprice.org

Group 2 Foods

Group 2 foods supply large quantities of essential vitamins and minerals. These include all organ meats, low fat fish, and shellfish. These foods are perfect to eat in smaller quantities, maybe 1-2 times per week. One of the ways I have found to get some of these super nutritious foods in my routine is to cut up frozen beef liver into small cubes and put them in my shakes. I am not a big fan of eating liver and have found this to be the best way to get it into my diet consistently without having to eat it directly. The quality and source of Group 2 food is also a significant factor. It is not always easy to find sources for properly caught fish. VitalChoice.com is a great resource to find the highest quality fish.

Group 3 Foods

Think of Group 3 foods as "Proceed with Caution". These are foods you want to eat sparingly and it will really depend on your tolerance levels. I know for me, eating too many grains, like bread, always has a negative effect on my Vitality Big 6. I am also half Italian so I love pizza. Eve and I will periodically fix homemade pizza using freshly made sourdough for the crust and add on all the fixings. In general, it's a good idea to monitor your reaction to these foods; as this will vary from person to person. The Group 3 foods that I completely avoid because of how my Big 6 responds are beans and legumes. I have found that some people, not many, have a little more tolerance for eating these things occasionally. I have not encountered many people who can eat beans and legumes regularly without being impacted by intestinal discomfort for all the reasons mentioned in chapter 5.

Group 4 Foods

In general, my rule is to avoid these foods as much as possible. The problem with many of the things in group four is that they are listed as an ingredient in almost every processed food, even when they are sold as organic. Artificial fats, cheap oils, and artificial sweeteners dominate our food supply. I would advise you to pick up everything you are thinking of purchasing at the grocery store and read the label carefully to make sure these substances are not in the ingredients. Sadly, just doing this simple ingredient check will eliminate about 80-90% of the foods in a grocery store.

Other Resources

If you would like some tools to help implement what you have learned including sample meal plan, balancing your macros, and some of our favorite recipes, visit www.healthtovitality. com/resources and download them for free!

Trilogy of Vitality Pillar II
Systemic Summary

➢ Five key variables to creating systemic vitality are
  1. Sleep
     a. 6-8 hours a night at a minimum
  2. Getting Outside
     a. The Perfect Breath: in for 6 seconds, out for 6 seconds
  3. Nutrition
  4. Mental-Emotional
  5. Movement
➢ Make your Vitality Big 6 the key reference point for systemic vitality and take into *consideration* the numbers on a blood test and the scale
➢ The best sources for your macronutrients:
  ○ Carbohydrates: Simple sugars like fruits, dairy, and tubers
  ○ Proteins: Animal protein like muscle meats, dairy, eggs, and broths
  ○ Fats: Saturated fats like coconut oil, butter, dairy, and beef
➢ The elimination of foods high in polyunsaturated fats will have the greatest impact on increasing vitality

TRILOGY OF VITALITY

PILLAR III: MINDSET

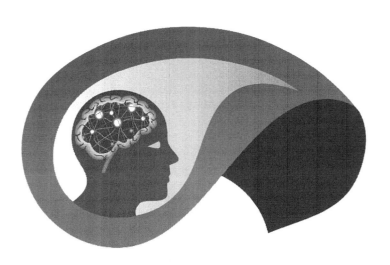

Chapter 7

IS YOUR MINDSET WORKING AGAINST YOUR BIOLOGY?

I got involved in the Self-Help/Personal Development world because I was on a journey to write about living a life of vitality and create the system that I am sharing with you in this book. I wanted to learn more about stress, mindset, psychology, and spirituality outside the context of religion in order to develop another set of tools and skills. This would not only help me manage the challenges in my own life but would also complete the Trilogy of Vitality I have now been working on for over twenty years. I believed this is where I would find everything I needed to create the third pillar that had been missing. Learning as much as I could in this area would allow me to work with all aspects of my clients' lives. It was time to take another deep dive!

The Global Self-Help industry was valued at over 41 billion dollars in 2021.[30] I have been engaged in it for the last ten years and have taken tens of thousands of dollars' worth of online courses from managing trauma to increasing

---

[30] Grand View Research (2018)

my productivity. I have been in a leadership position with one company for about seven of those years. One thing I can tell you after being involved for so long is that most of these organizations have good intentions, but some are primarily focused on building their own fame, wealth, and position in the industry. I can confidently say a lot of them are using frameworks and techniques that are intended to create dependency, just as the fitness, movement, systemic health, and nutrition professions have done.

There are thousands of people who will tell you they have benefited tremendously from these organizations, and I'm not debating this. However, many who have benefited have done so at a price that I will be discussing later in this chapter. Thousands of people have spent tens of thousands of dollars on programs, seminars, and memberships that promise them they will be "fixed," live up to their potential and finally "be enough"- only to keep finding themselves in a similar position to the one they started in. They never "get there" and are worse off as a result. I had to ask myself, with all of the billions of dollars that are being spent on personal development, why are so many people suffering from so many mental illnesses and becoming more dependent on modalities, treatments, and medications than ever before?

Is the whole personal development industry one big conspiracy? Of course not! But you do have to remember it's run by people who are floating around in the realm of subjectivity. When that subjectivity is left to be interpreted and defined by just a single leader or guru - things tend to go south. The requirements for acceptance, approval, and inclusion can become rigid, divisive, and unbalanced and are based almost entirely on what has worked for this one person, what that person's limitations are, and what their own personal goal is.

One of the ways some of the leaders run these organizations is to use simple frameworks that inappropriately or inaccurately mix good applications of psychology with their personal agenda. This may lead them to ask you to focus on creating goals and a lifestyle that will become a lifelong inner battle for you. The worst part of this inner battle is that it is one you cannot win. I know this from first hand experience.

Keep in mind that when I got involved in this self-help, personal development world, I had already developed two of the three pillars of my own system by deep diving into the systems that were traditionally used in those fields. As a result, I had consistently discovered that very few of them were based on the most effective and natural methods that were compatible with how our bodies were designed to work best. They were based on systems that kept people needing the product or service indefinitely. As I got more deeply engaged, I found I was expected to set aside my own knowledge, understanding, training, skills, experience, and desires in favor of using just one approach to help people in all areas. Because I was committed to learning everything I could and I trusted my mentor, I did my very best, unsuccessfully, to buy into this idea. However hard I tried to ignore it, there were increasingly strong intuitive and biological communications telling me something was seriously off. I also was continuously told to fight the urge to support people with their physical ailments and systemic needs because it didn't align with the organization's agenda. I felt trapped in this internal battle I couldn't seem to win.

Now my example may be an extreme one— to feel as if I were in an all-out war with myself. However, it is important to realize that when you are constantly fighting battles inside yourself you can develop habits of self-doubt and end up not trusting yourself. Eventually, this will cause a disconnection between yourself and your emotional communication systems. Your emotional communication system gives you feedback for your behavior and lets you know if it is damaging or helpful. If this dissociation becomes too severe it can lead to personality disorders. What allowed me to actually win this internal war were the emotions of anger and frustration I kept feeling. It is always important to ask what an emotion is trying to communicate to you, which is exactly what I was being told *not* to do. My emotional communication system, which I will discuss further in this chapter, finally broke through and forced me to listen after trying to communicate with me for years.

I finally realized that my anger and frustration were giving me very important information. Not only was it time for me to move on and finish designing my own program, my feelings were pinpointing the areas where what I was trying to learn went against what my biology was telling me. I realized that these disjunctions I was experiencing were very important areas of me to address in my third pillar.

Some self-help programs leverage techniques that sell you on the idea that you need to stay involved forever. Some will even promote them as the path to mastery, which conveniently is very supportive of their business model. In this next chapter we will be looking at the three main concepts existing in the mindset arena that pit us directly against our biology. They are:

1. Pursuing happiness or other positive emotions as a goal
2. Believing that "Negative emotions" are an obstacle to be overcome
3. Avoiding and mitigating stress

The Danger of Pursuing Happiness

Let's start with this idea that our goal should be to focus on pursuing happiness or other emotions like joy, peace, and freedom. On top of this goal, there is the idea that happiness is a choice and that your internal experience is something you can choose regardless of the environment. If you are not happy and fulfilled at work, you are told it's because you have a pattern of being dissatisfied. If you are looking for your job to fulfill you (or anything else for that matter) and it doesn't, then you are doing it wrong and need to *work harder* on yourself. I have seen too many people, including myself, stick around unhealthy environments trying to convince themselves that if they just worked harder on themselves, they could be happy and fulfilled. This is an example of one of those losing battles.

One of the top things people tell me when beginning as a coaching client is they just want to be at peace. Now I'm not saying that this isn't what they want at that moment, but I can tell you for sure, it isn't their desired final destination. I usually walk these clients through a thought exercise where I have them imagine that all their problems have magically disappeared. All their stresses and stressors are gone and they are finally at peace. And then I ask them, "Now that you are at peace, what would you do?" More often than not they say, "Nothing, I'd do nothing." And I absolutely believe this is a real and authentic answer at that moment—but it is also usually a sign they are burned out, exhausted, and need a break. My follow up question is, "OK, so after you do nothing, then what are you going to do? Because you can only sit around in a hammock on the beach for so long before it gets *really* boring." This usually gets them thinking about what they would do if they really could do anything. If they eliminated all the *have-tos* and perceived burdens in their lives, what would be possible? The previously inconceivable answers often start as simple, seemingly small things like: I'd read a book about "x", I'd go hiking, I'd take a trip to Italy, I'd learn how to play an instrument, or I'd go back to school. All these answers are the seedlings to what is truly meaningful and important to that individual, which is actually the destination they are seeking.

Another example of this idea of an emotion being the goal is expressed by the individuals who want to "know FREEDOM!" These individuals sprint to retirement day because not having a job means they will finally "know freedom!" They believe "knowing freedom" is their goal because they can finally stop working and that means they can get up whenever they want, not have to answer to anyone, and do whatever they want all day. They are finally free to choose how they spend their time and resources. What commonly happens in this scenario? Feelings, not of freedom, but of restlessness and the need to find something to do. More often than not, it is to find something that is meaningful to them. Something that is super important and needs them to invest a lot of their attention. Some examples of these activities include golf, knitting, quilting, volunteer work, model building, studying, travel and even mentoring younger generations.

One of the first goals I set when I was completely overworked, working six and a half days a week, was to have Saturdays completely free—a day when I could sleep until my body naturally woke up. A day where I had no work responsibilities and I could do what I wanted to do the entire day. I could hang with the family, sit on the couch, chill, and just enjoy life! Pure and utter freedom was the target. I remember busting my butt to make that happen. I reorganized my schedule making sure the clients and work responsibilities were covered and arriving at the time when Saturday was completely free. That first Saturday was magical. I slept until I woke up, came downstairs, ate breakfast with the family, sat on the couch and relaxed. It was great. I had arrived at happiness and freedom! Well, let's just say that didn't last very long. After a few Saturdays of relaxing, I started getting very restless. It got so bad that I became irritable. I was so irritable that at one point Eve told me if I was just going to be cranky all day, I should go back to the office and work. This was really confusing to me. I had finally reached the final destination called freedom, peace, and happiness—why was I such a cranky beast?

Although there was some short-term relief in actually having a day off, until I created a meaning and a purpose for that day, real freedom, happiness, and fulfillment were not available to me.

Unfortunately, all of what I have just shared, isn't even the real downside of the pursue-positive-emotion framework. I found pursuing happiness to be one of the most destructive frameworks in personal development. Because the focus is on feeling good (happy) emotions, it creates conflict when we are feeling bad emotions. This conflict can manifest in a few ways. When feeling good emotions is the goal, then we will do everything we can to avoid feeling the bad emotions, because who wants to do things wrong? One way people manage this is by denying they have negative emotions and convincing themselves they don't get angry or don't get resentful, especially when facing the public. They portray the image that their life is just full of peace, joy, and happiness.

Social media makes this a much easier image to uphold and portray. We see examples of this facade being shattered on a regular basis when a public figure is being exposed for their hypocrisy. Whether it is someone that publicly stands against drugs while being a closet addict or someone who publically vilifies sexual harassment and is accused of sexual harassment by countless employees. The reality is that nobody can sustainably suppress and deny these naturally occurring emotional states and cover them with over-exaggerated positivity. When someone covers up these negative emotions and denies their presence, sooner or later the emotions build up and come out in explosive ways, express themselves through destructive behaviors, or manifest as disease over time. Over-exaggerated positivity is called "toxic positivity" and it is not only toxic to the person doing it, it is also toxic to be around.

Fortunately and unfortunately I have had first-hand experience doing this to myself, engaging with individuals and communities who promote this, and have coached many individuals who portray this image publicly and struggle tremendously behind the scenes. As they fight to keep their positive image going with toxic positivity, they are constantly beating themselves up for feeling these negative emotions and demanding of themselves that these patterns of negative emotions be eliminated. They relate to these emotions as a sign of weakness and believe that there is something wrong with them if they are unable to eliminate or "let them go". Conveniently, some personal development organizations and groups have "special" programs costing thousands of dollars that people are encouraged to go to multiple times, to attempt to get these "toxic" and "destructive patterns" removed.

In these extreme cases, where there is intense focus around "removing destructive patterns", there is a complete dissociation that happens from all these feelings, which is by far the most dangerous. When you dissociate from your emotional communication system, you have no inner barometer or feedback system for your behaviors and actions, and you are able to justify *any* action you take—no matter how destructive or damaging it may be. Someone who is completely dissociated from their emotions and has no empathy for others or the world is what is considered to be borderline sociopathic.

The bottom line? The approach of pursuing happiness or any positive emotional state as the end game goes directly against the biological purpose of our emotions. Because of this, we will not only be working on ourselves forever, but we will be working against ourselves forever.

The Biological Purpose of Emotions

It's time to think about emotions differently. To begin with, it is important to define the concept and idea of emotions and their purpose clearly. Although there is no universally accepted definition of emotion, one of the easiest ways to think of emotions is inside of two spectrums: energetic and affect. The energetic spectrum ranges from low energy to high energy. The *affect side* ranges from feelings that are pleasant to feelings that are unpleasant. This can sound like "I feel tired (energy) but content (affect)".

The Yale Center for Emotional Intelligence created "The Mood Meter," an app that trains emotional awareness and sensitivity. I have found it to be a good resource if you'd like to get more in touch with your emotions. It uses these two spectrums to help pinpoint the specific emotion you may be feeling at any given time.

But what I want to really focus on in this section is the *role* of emotions, because this is where I have seen the greatest area of confusion. A common theme that I see in the self help and psychological disciplines is the villainization of emotions, making them something to eliminate, tolerate, and/or mitigate. Although the newer approach of accepting and "letting them go" is better than ignoring or stomaching emotions, it is actually still missing the mark on understanding and leveraging emotional communication. Looking at emotions as destructive in any way is not helpful. It is time to acknowledge and treat emotions as valuable allies and friends. They have the ability to convey a lot of information to us in a very short period of time. Communicating information to us quickly and efficiently is their primary role and is essential to surviving and thriving. An example of this can be feelings of danger and uncertainty. This communication can be instantaneous so we can quickly take action to lead us to safety. Many times, we may not even be able to explain why we left, but "something" told us to get out of there. That "something" is our emotions.

Emotions are communicating to us at all times. They are communicating whether or not we are aligned with something that is important, meaningful, or of value to us. It is similar to a navigation system that tells you what direction you are heading in. When you put a destination in your navigation application, the goal isn't for the app to talk to you nicely and make you feel good. It is there to tell you if you are heading in the right or wrong direction. It's function is to ensure you get to your destination. This is exactly the purpose of emotions. Although emotional communication can be intricate and complex, at a very basic level, when you feel a *negative* emotion, it is a communication that there is something you need to pay attention to and that an adjustment may be needed, sometimes immediately. When you feel a *positive* emotion, it is most likely communicating to you that you are on track and to stay the course. For all of these reasons, it is important to understand and acknowledge that it is impossible *not* to have negative emotions.

If we are primarily focused on having a certain type of emotional experience like joy, peace, and happiness, then we are not focused on any particular destination. You may be saying, "but wait, what if being happy and peaceful is the destination I want to reach?" I would say happiness may be the experience you'd like to have on the journey or when you reach your goal, but feeling/experiencing the emotion of joy isn't your ultimate destination. My colleague, Josh Guerrero, with whom I created the *Arena Method Courses*, had a great analogy to demonstrate this concept. If you had an IV drip that immediately made you happy and peaceful and you didn't have to do anything but just sit there forever feeling happy and peaceful, would you do it? The catch is, you could not pursue anything, connect with people, learn, grow, make an impact in the world, nothing—but happiness and peace would be guaranteed. My guess is you would not opt in for the IV. I would bet that you would much rather pursue and reach a destination that has value and is meaningful to you. A destination that has you connecting with people you love, learning, growing, exploring, and creating an impact in the world. You'd choose that even if it meant there would be times of non-happiness and even stress. This then begs the question, why would someone pursue something that might elicit challenges, hardship, and moments of negative emotion? We do it because it's worth it and is intrinsically meaningful. This shifts the focus away from pursuing an "emotional state" and onto a worthy pursuit.

It's how this stress is handled that allows you to fulfill what is most meaningful. In the next section, you will see how stress is also a communication, similar to our emotions, and how trying to mitigate and avoid it, is very destructive.

Why You Should Not Try To Manage, Mitigate, Or Avoid Stress

One of the questions I asked every mentor, doctor, and health practitioner I ever studied with was how they defined stress. The vast variety of responses I received fascinated me. Some couldn't define it, others articulated what created it, like traffic, money, or kids, and some gave some abstract answers. It quickly became apparent, that this was a relatively ambiguous and subjective topic. Over twenty years of exploring this question, working with thousands of individuals in an intimate way in the space of body mechanics, systemic support, and the mental/emotional space, I landed on a way to relate to stress by defining it relative to the three components of vitality—physical, systemic, and mental.

Physical stress is often the easiest to identify. It can be viewed as a biomechanical stress to the system that can have different effects. The forces that act on the body naturally, like gravity, ground reaction forces, mass, momentum, and so on, place stress on the physical body every day. Physical stress can also be caused by acute impact, like getting hit in the shin by a baseball, stubbing your toe on the coffee table, or banging your knee on the ground. Physical stress can be leveraged for growth or can create injury.

Systemic stress can be defined as the moment the body activates a series of events commonly referred to as the "stress response" that increases biological resources to take action, and in some cases, massive action. The body's stress response secretes the hormones of adrenaline and cortisol which increase heart rate and blood pressure to provide the energetic resources to address whatever the "stressful" situation is. An example might be when you are awakened from a sound sleep by an explosion nearby, pop up out of bed, and are ready to take massive action. Then you find out the frightening noise was caused by a neighbor setting off fireworks and there is no danger. Now you have to deal with the stress response and figure out how to calm down and go back to sleep.

The final definition is the state of <u>mental or emotional stress</u>. This is one of the more important definitions because it directly correlates and speaks to the "X-Factor" that I mentioned in chapter 1. Stanford professor and decorated researcher, Alia Crum, defines stress in the following way:

> *"The experience or anticipation of adversity in our goal-related efforts"*[31]

I find this definition fascinating and very telling. There is a condition of stress built into this definition. The condition is having goal-related efforts or something we want. If I were to ask you if you were stressed out when the Boston Celtics were up two games to one against the Golden State Warriors in the 2022 NBA Finals, you would have one of three answers. Yes—super stressed, no—I was excited, or no—I didn't care who won. So, what is the *key* variable that must be in place in order for any of us to be mentally and emotionally stressed? It has to be something that is important or meaningful to us; we have to care about the outcome.

The only way something can cause you stress is if you care about that something. This means that the only real way to eliminate stress is to stop caring! And I bet you have had moments where something was so stressful and you felt so helpless to do anything about it, that you did just stop caring. This is a very effective strategy to eliminate stress. There are people I know who have taken this approach to life in general. They just stopped caring about anything. This is usually the last resort in managing stress.

---

[31] Crum Alia and Lyddy Cris (2013)

It follows then that the only way to mitigate, avoid, or manage stress is to do our best to mitigate, avoid, or manage the caring. This can look like managing stress by meditating, working out, eating healthy food, going to church, doing focused breathing, going on retreats, and so on. All of these things have a place and be helpful, but not as a way to avoid things that most likely need to be addressed. In the personal development space the idea of acceptance to mitigate stress is popular. Meaning, you acknowledge you are "stressed", feel and accept that it is there, do a few belly breaths, and "let it go". However, I found many times that acceptance, when applied in this context, became a way to numb oneself. A major downside to acceptance in this manner is that it dampens the motivation system to take action when something is not OK. If I eliminate the caring, I eliminate the drive to act.

There is absolutely a place for acceptance, but when taken to extremes to eliminate stress, it creates apathy and disconnection. Once again, trying to eliminate or mitigate stress has us working against ourselves, creating massive inner conflicts.

Part of my own experience in the personal development space was that I found myself muscling myself to accept and almost numbing myself to things that I would have been upset about normally. In the short term it was wonderful, because it eliminated the immediate discomfort of the stress. But this stress communication, like emotional communication, is not something that can be eliminated and will build up over time. Later in this chapter, I will discuss how to align and partner with stress so we can leverage our biology to support us on our journey.

Align Your Mindset with Your Biology

Pursue Meaning Not Happiness

When I think of my journey to find answers and create a framework that gave me access to the kind of vitality and meaning I wanted to experience, I am amazed at what I was able to navigate and overcome. The failures, hardships, challenges, and obstacles that showed up along the way were things that I could never have imagined being able to deal with. I remember a pivotal moment that inspired me to double down on my commitment to pursue my purpose to find the path to vitality. It came at a point when I was about to give up. I was listening to a Tim Ferris podcast during one of the many hours I spent in my car on Los Angeles freeways. The title of the podcast was "The Man Who Studied 1,000 Deaths to Learn How to Live." The podcast guest was BJ Miller, who is known as an "expert in death" due to his work interviewing and spending time with over 1,000 people at the end of their lives. He caught these individuals at a time of deep reflection on their life's journey. He revealed the biggest regrets these individuals had as they neared the end. There were the usual ones, of course, like wishing they had spent more time with family and friends, but the one that had the greatest impact on me was a little different. The number one regret these individuals had was not "going for it." They were left wondering what their life would have looked like had they had the courage to pursue the thing in which they were most interested and that held the most meaning for them.

While hearing this author articulate the pain he perceived these individuals were in during this realization, I felt it throughout my whole being. It immediately became the thing I feared most. At that moment, I committed myself to "going for it", to not be at the end of my life regretting the fact that I hadn't followed my dream. And if it weren't for that commitment, I would never have had the experience and impact of starting my clinic in Los Angeles, creating and teaching online courses for the last ten years, and I certainly would not have written this book.

So how do we position ourselves to leverage the power of our emotional communication system? The way to align and leverage this incredibly powerful tool is to get super clear on what is most meaningful and important for us to fulfill in our lives. This could be in reference to the immediate future or the next twenty-plus years. The goal we have as humans is not to live a happy life, it is to live a meaningful and purposeful life. When we are living a meaningful and purposeful life, the by-product is fulfillment, joy, peace and happiness.

The work of Viktor Frankl, the author of *Man's Search for Meaning* and a survivor of 4 Nazi concentration camps, illustrated and demonstrated the power of identifying and naming a meaning and purpose for life. He developed the idea of logotherapy.[32] *Logos* is Greek for "meaning" and logotherapy is a mindset that focuses on the meaning of human existence. It is built on the principle that not only are humans motivated by meaning but their resiliency and tolerance to overcome obstacles is directly correlated to the strength of this meaning.

"He who has a Why to live for can bear almost any How."[33]
—*Frederick Nietzche*

Think about a time in your life when you felt a high-level fulfillment, wholeness, and peace within yourself. I'll

---

[32] Frankl Viktor (2006)
[33] Nietzsche Friedrich (1998)

bet it was after you accomplished something very important, and I wouldn't be surprised if it was accompanied by some challenges and struggles. Our resiliency to achieve and overcome anything that life can throw at us is amplified and optimized when we are pursuing something that is mission-critical to us. Some examples of this are completing a college degree or Ph.D. program, getting in shape for a wedding, getting the job we want, or winning a competition or event. We tie a high amount of value to these things.

Our visions and pursuits, especially if they are lofty, come with their share of hardships, challenges, and obstacles, but the thing that has us persevere and optimize our human potential is the meaning and purpose we attach to fulfilling the outcomes.

Now let me be clear, this is not the path most traveled, and society is not set up to support and champion us on this journey. Our society is set up to distract us, like the sirens of Greek mythology, with enticing songs promising temporary relief of discomfort and delivering short-term pleasures. Aligning and committing to living a meaningful and purposeful life is hard. Not only do we have to learn how to resist the calling sirens of contemporary society but there are also going to be dragons to slay. But I can tell you with absolute certainty—it is totally worth it.

Before we start the process of focusing on the pursuit of meaning in your life, let us first understand what is most meaningful to our biology. There are certain things that are hard wired into our operating system that direct and govern our decision making, whether we are aware of them or not. It is essential to understand these biological drivers and learn to align them appropriately, if we truly want to be in the driver's seat of our life experience.

Understand What is Most Meaningful
to Your Biology First

There are only two things your evolutionary biology
cares about when it comes to what is most important and
meaningful. Those two things are safety and belonging. If
we don't perceive we are safe or accepted, everything else
is irrelevant. These two mechanisms are what have the
greatest impact on our ability to self-regulate. The ability to
self-regulate is one of the most fundamental human needs.
Self-regulation is the ability to turn off and direct the stress
response in a positive and productive way.

Abraham Maslow was the first to put a framework
around what is most important and meaningful with his
Hierarchy of Needs Pyramid[34] (Fig 35). At the bottom of
his pyramid, the most foundational need is safety and
physiological needs. This is survival biology and it drives
everything. When you look at the brain, you can break it
down into two general categories, the new brain and the old
brain. The new brain is what is referred to as the neocortex
and is responsible for critical thinking, problem-solving, and
creating frameworks, perspectives, and belief structures. The
old brain consists of everything else, like the brain stem,
midbrain, and limbic system. The old brain is the part of
the brain that is responsible for keeping us alive and governs
basic processes like breathing, heart rate, digestion, etc.—
things that are essential to the survival of the body. Old brain
activity processes take precedence over everything else. When
these basic needs are not met, everything else takes a back
seat. These foundational physiological needs are the primary
ways the system creates safety.

---

[34] Maslow Abraham (1943)

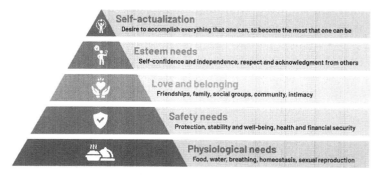

Fig 36: Maslow's Hierarchy of Meaning

Another way our system determines what is safe and what is not is by constantly evaluating what is familiar to us and what is not. This is the base of Maslow's hierarchy in action. Familiarity equates to safety. If we are used to being treated poorly or not valued, then our brain associates that familiar environment as a safe environment even though it is unpleasant. If we were exposed to environments where we were valued as who we are, then that becomes the familiar environment. In this case we would have an affinity for environments that value and respect us.

Our brain and nervous system operate like a prediction machine and want to accurately predict things. This is why the brain seeks and has an affinity to find and exist in environments it knows. In familiar environments, it can accurately predict things. It has expectations of how the world looks and finds comfort when the world matches those expectations, it feels safe and secure. It wants the world to be predictable. How many times have you, or someone you know, engaged with someone who was untruthful, knowing they were untruthful? When they eventually lie or betray you, you proudly declare, "I knew they were going to do that," as if your prediction was a badge of honor. In a weird way you feel better about it because you knew it was going to happen, even though it doesn't feel good and is not what you want in a relationship.

This phenomenon was also illustrated by the success of a popular children's TV show called *Blue's Clues*. This show was the first to discover that kids find comfort in knowing what is coming. *Blue's Clues* was the first children's TV program that replayed the same episode every day for a week at a time. They found great success with this strategy because kids engaged every day, even though it was the same episode. For all you parents out there, this explains why you may have watched Disney's *Frozen* about three hundred times with your child. The mechanism that is looking to regulate the system by matching predictions with reality is what made Blue's Clues the popular kids' show that it became.

This same mechanism will unconsciously drive you to be attracted to and simultaneously attract to you, environments, people, and things that align with past experiences. This could be a problem when past experiences are not the experiences you are looking to create, especially when these experiences are painful or dangerous.

There is, however, an aspect that is important to understand that also lives in this foundational need category, and it is something that happens as soon as we are born. It is a mechanism that is biologically activated to ensure survival and it is called the attachment drive.[35] When we are born, the attachment drive immediately seeks to attach to someone in the environment to ensure survival. Human offspring are not only the most dependent species, but we are also dependent for the longest period of time. We *need* the people and caregivers in our environment to take care of us for our survival. We are completely dependent on others to keep us alive. The attachment drive helps us attach to one of

---

[35] Wikipedia. "Attachment Theory." (2022)

the caregivers to ensure they take care of us. In the book *Hold on to Your Kids*,[36] Gabor Maté, M.D. and Gordan Neufield, Ph.D. identify six ways of attaching:

1. Senses—physical touch
2. Sameness—mimicking the adults in the environment
3. Belonging and Loyalty—accepted by the environment
4. Significance—we matter and are important
5. Feeling—to crave and know love
6. Being Known—being seen and heard

These six ways of attaching not only ensure survival, but when they are met they allow the system to be self-regulated and relaxed. When any of these things are threatened, the system is stressed, in a state of anxiety, and many times panicked.

One of the most telling examples of this is the Still Face Experiment by Dr. Edward Tronick.[37] In this experiment, Dr. Tronick demonstrates the stress an infant, around the age of one year old, experiences when it senses a disconnection to its mother. The experiment starts with the mother engaging with her infant through touch, sounds, loving expressions, and overall acknowledgement. Then the mother is instructed to just simply sit there with a "still face" while looking at the infant, but no longer engaging. The response of the infant is fascinating. You can see the infant start to look confused as if she isn't sure what's happening. She makes some attempts to get the connection back by smiling, pointing, and gesturing in different ways. When that doesn't work, you can see

---

[36] Maté Gabor and Neufeld Gordon (2006)
[37] Tronick Edward (1975)

some anxiety emerge as she starts to fuss and make louder screeching sounds hoping to regain her mom's engagement. And finally after all of these failed attempts, she begins to almost give up and look away and enter a visible state of stress and irritation. Every part of that infant's instincts to self-regulate and be calm and relaxed, is dependent on the connection to its caregiver. It is a very powerful video that still hurts my heart to watch.

In addition to this need for attachment, there is another basic human need we have—the ability to be authentic. Authenticity is the ability to both be aware of what we are feeling and have the freedom to express it. It is biologically essential for us to be connected to what we are feeling. Being aware of what we are feeling can be the difference between life and death. Our emotions, as I mentioned in the earlier section, are communication systems that inform us what is happening at any moment. And one of the things they communicate is danger. If we are unable to hear the signals communicating danger, we are in big trouble.

The important thing to note and understand is that when we are children, the need to be accepted supersedes the need to be authentic. This means that we will disconnect from our feelings, our needs, and our authentic expression in order to be accepted by the environment. When we are children it is absolutely essential that we get our environment to accept us. If the environment does not accept us and take care of us, then we are on our own, and no infant or young child is able to keep themselves alive. This puts the child in a position of needing to create versions of themselves that are accepted by their environment even when this means putting their feelings and needs aside and taking on an acceptable persona. Suppressing our need to be authentic can manifest when we assume roles like taking care of everyone else, being the "good kid", the athletic one, the smart one, the peacemaker, the quiet one, or as Dr. Gabor Mate puts it, we embody super autonomous self sufficiency.

These versions of ourselves that we develop in order to be accepted by the environment are what I refer to as our adapted selves. An adapted self is a version of us that we create in order to get the environment to accept us—to feel like we belong. The need to belong is hard-wired in the old brain and is directly tied to our ability to survive. As we evolved as human beings, we survived by sticking together, focusing on putting community first. No one individual was more important than the whole. If you were not accepted by your community, it most likely meant death. There was a time when the most severe penalty or sentence someone could receive wasn't death, it was exile. The Romans specifically had elaborate laws around exile and banishment. There were essentially two options, "fuga" and banishment. *Fuga* was voluntary exile or flight, and banishment was forced exile. They even had four levels of banishment that varied in severity of duration and location.[38]

Clearly we don't have these laws in our society today, but the drive to not be separated from the herd or our tribe is still prevalent. Today this manifests as the need to fit in with groups of friends, colleagues, or communities. I'm sure you can think of a time when you sacrificed your authentic needs and wants in order to please someone else or to fit in with a group of friends. This is something we can all relate to because of that biologically-driven care about what people think of us. The key to leveraging this drive is to know who we want to authentically be, learn to decipher who the individuals and communities are who align with who we want to be authentically, and figure out how to align our need to be accepted with groups that match us. You do this

---

[38]   Ovid and the Censored Voice (2022)

by having a clear vision of who you want to be and the kind of people with whom you want to be connected. Once you know what is most important to you and you have clarity and have named your values, it's time to seek out individuals and communities that vibrate and resonate with these values. This is where you should care what they think. If they are embodying the way of being that is authentically most important to you, then it is healthy and very supportive to care what they think and use them as a barometer to make necessary calibrations in your own life to ensure you are aligned with who you want to be.

The applications of these calibrations depend on the context, but one simple example of this would be in the case where someone is teaching you a skill that you are interested in learning. When I was learning how to evaluate human movement, pinpoint root causes of people's mechanical pain, and design a strategy to help them, I cared very much about what my mentor thought about what I was doing. I wanted him to approve of my thought process and approach because I was interested in building the capacity he had.

Where it gets a little hairy and where we must be very careful, is when we have not taken the time to get clear on who and what is most important to us and we allow our adapted self to select who and what is important. In my example with my mentor, I had a very clear vision of what was important for me to learn. If this is not the case, there is a good chance that our adapted self will take over. Remember, our adapted self is the version of ourselves that we created as children when we *needed* the environment to accept us. A child relates to its environment as the world, because its environment at that time does make up the entirety of a child's world. Our psyche translates this to needing the world to accept us. If we have not clearly and consciously identified who and what we want to become, the default selection the brain will choose is, get "the world" to accept and like us. As some of us know first hand, there is nothing more exhausting, lonely, and defeating than trying to get everyone else's approval for how we live our lives.

There was a time in my life when this need to have the world accept me and like me became extremely destructive. It was when I was running my clinic in Los Angeles. I had a very hard time saying no to anyone who asked for my help even if I was exhausted, overworked, and absolutely did not want to do it. I scheduled people during my lunch break, early in the morning, on weekends - whenever. If someone was in need, I threw on my superhero cape and came to the rescue! Yes, one of my adapted selves was a superhero, and he caused me a lot of grief. The result of this was being completely overwhelmed and overburdened, trying to take care of everyone. It then manifested into feeling a lot of resentment for everyone who needed my help, which then made me feel guilty for resenting them.

If these basic biological needs for attachment and authenticity are not properly integrated as we move into our adult years, suffering is inevitable and in the worst-case scenario, we become very disconnected from ourselves. At best, we experience a low level of anxiety, restlessness, and emptiness inside accompanied by feelings of never being enough. At worst, we develop very destructive habits and relationships in our lives.

If we do not properly integrate these core biological needs of attachment and authenticity then the option that remains is to manage, cope, and numb ourselves with a variety of modalities. Alcohol, drugs (prescription and non-prescription), food, scrolling social media, watching hours of TV, retail therapy, and affairs are a few of the more common ones. All of these are strategies to self-regulate, to take the edge off, to feel alive, to feel significant, to feel accepted, or feel safe.

The ALIGN Online Course that I created is designed to walk you through all of these concepts and integrate them into your life in a seamless way. For more information on ALIGN, go to www.healthtovitality.com/align.

Leveraging your Most Powerful Communication System

One of the most important biological systems to learn how to work with is our stress response. It is also one of the most misunderstood biological responses. One of the top reasons people come to me is because they are looking for help on how to mitigate, manage, or eliminate stress. By the time they have come to me, many have already tried countless techniques and modalities. Before we get into a different way to manage stress, let's review and expand on our working definition of stress. Alia Crum's definition of stress from earlier in this chapter was,

"The experience or anticipation of adversity in our goal-related efforts" [39]

The "experience" she is referring to is emotion. When I am stressed or when I engage with someone who is stressed, one common thing is always present— emotions like overwhelm, fear, sadness, anxiety, insecurity, hopelessness, and self-doubt. And these emotions are usually associated with a threat of adversity interfering with something that we care about. The old way of dealing with these emotions

---

[39] Crum Alia and Lyddy Chris (2013)

would be to suppress, distract, or repress them. The newer way is to accept the emotions, breathe through them, and let them pass. Both of these approaches can be helpful in the short term, but are not ideal and cause long-term problems.

Suppression, denial, and distraction are not generally accepted as great options because of the long-term implications of suppressing emotion. This strategy manifests itself through emotional outbursts, projecting these emotions onto others, and eventually disease. When I was in the throes of my overwhelm, working six and half days a week at my clinic in Los Angeles as my superhero-adapted self, I could control that overwhelm and frustration at work, for the most part, but it sure did come out when I was home. My lack of patience and short fuse was evident with Eve and the kids. I was always operating at the edge and had very little tolerance. Not only was this impacting my relationships but it was also impacting my health. I was bloated, suffered from headaches, had trouble sleeping, and was walking a fine line with my high blood pressure levels. If you ask any physician what the most significant contributor to poor health is, stress will be at the top of the list.

The good news was that I had started learning a new way to manage my emotions. I was beginning to become aware and acknowledge what I was feeling, accept it, breathe through it, and let it go. Now, this is definitely a better strategy than denying and suppressing, but it still didn't get me to my optimal outcome of vitality. Although it helped me in the short term, in the long term it was something I had to do all day long. It helped in the moments the emotions arose, but they didn't stop coming. This was the beginning of that battle that started to ignite inside me. I felt like I was constantly breathing and letting go of the emotion. Turns out, there is no such thing as letting go of an emotion, but we will address that later in this chapter.

If you remember from earlier in the book, we defined the role of emotions as a communication system. Acknowledging and accepting the emotion that is present is definitely a step in the right direction. However, the step that is essential (and often missed) is the "integration" of that communication. It is very important to ask what this emotion is trying to communicate, and then make sure to integrate or apply the information that it is providing you, similar to a GPS. What good is it, if our GPS tells us to turn right, we hear and acknowledge it, but never actually turn the steering wheel to the right? I wish I could tell you there are universal communications for each emotion, but that has not been identified. Like most things in life, it depends on the situation and context to determine what the emotion may be communicating. The table below illustrates a few examples of what an emotion may be communicating in different scenarios and contexts:

Context	Emotion	Potential Communication	Step to Integration
Starting a new job or venture	Self-Doubt and Anxiety	Pay attention: You are about to engage in something you know little to nothing about. You may not be equipped to manage what is coming.	Owning that this is true and taking some steps to better equip yourself for the new venture can ensure that you will be successful
Friend says they are going to do something for you, and they don't do it	Frustration and Anger	Pay Attention: The expectations we have with this individual may not align with the capacity of the individual.	Assess the capacity of the individual and either calibrate the expectation or bring the expectation to someone that is capable of meeting it
A loved one is leaving that you haven't seen in a long time	Sadness	Pay Attention: These types of relationships are really important to you and you deeply care about these types of experiences You tie great meaning to these interactions	Make a conscious effort to create time for more of these types of relationships and interactions in your life

When you start to look at emotions in the above context you will realize how beneficial ALL emotions are to help us navigate through life. With this insight, emotions now become an asset instead of some inconvenience to manage.

One of the places where this can be more intricate and complicated is in situations where we have suppressed certain emotions from our past and therefore never integrated the communication. There are good reasons why emotions were suppressed and integration was not an option. One of the main reasons for this is an unsafe environment, especially if it happened in our childhood. An example of this is a child who grew up in an environment where its caregivers were overwhelmed by the things they were trying to manage in their lives, and were therefore unable to manage or tolerate a child's needs and experiences.

My example of my overwhelming experience with my clinic is a perfect one. When I came home completely overwhelmed and exhausted, and Christian or Emma were authentically expressing an emotion of excitement, sadness or disappointment about something, I had no capacity to manage it, so I would not engage with them. A child quickly learns they have to suppress those authentic emotional expressions if they want to connect with their caregiver. My children realized at some point that too much emotional expression would inhibit their connection to me at that moment. So if Christian and Emma wanted to connect with me when I was frustrated, they'd have to suppress some of their feelings. For many children, expressing their feelings and needs was not something that was welcomed in their environment, and in many cases threatened their acceptance by their environment. In these cases, the only option was to suppress, disconnect, and numb the emotions which meant the communication never came through and it certainly wasn't integrated.

As you can see, being able to disconnect from our emotions at the moment has its value - but that is not to say that it doesn't come with a host of long-term side effects, if we don't revisit, feel, and properly integrate those emotional experiences, they will haunt us forever. When these emotional communications we felt as children never get a chance to express, the communication system continues to try to feel, express, and communicate the information until it is heard and integrated—and there is no timeline for it to expire. It's important to remember that the emotional communication system is governed by the old brain and the old brain has no awareness of time. If you recall, the old brain is the part of the brain that governs survival and is different from the new brain that is rational and able to think critically about things. The old brain gets locked into needing to express the authentic feelings that were felt at eight years old. The more often this happens, the more feelings that are suppressed, the more powerful they become. Therefore, a forty-five-year-old adult may still get the communications of an eight-year-old child because they were never properly acknowledged and integrated. This explains why so many adults behave and respond like children, especially when certain emotions have never found expression. This gets very dangerous when these adults, behaving like children, have resources and power to amplify their temper tantrums and create more destruction than simply throwing themselves on the floor screaming and yelling. Just take a look at some of the world leaders today— quite scary actually.

In these cases, there is a benefit to going into the past to properly integrate certain experiences. Be cautious, though, of getting caught in the past, or it may become a cross to bear for the rest of your life. Talking about the past for years and years is an indication that communication has not been integrated in a constructive way.

Gabor Maté, a world renowned trauma specialist, defines trauma as not what happened to you, but as what happened *in you* as a result of what happened to you.[40] This is a very important distinction because you can't change what happened, but you can change how you relate to what happened. One of the main ways you can change how you relate to what happened is by acknowledging and integrating the emotional communication that was occurring inside.

The flow chart, on the next page, is a framework for integrating emotional communication from the ALIGN courses that I developed.(Fig 37). The framework is modeled after the work of Gabor Maté and his method of Compassionate Inquiry. As described on his website, "Compassionate Inquiry® is a psychotherapeutic approach that reveals what lies beneath the appearance we present to the world."[41] It's about getting to know yourself and understanding why you are the way you are, accepting it, and finding its place in your life today. The purpose of this work is not to let go of your trauma, fix yourself, or any variation of those things. It is to create a seamless tapestry of your life by finding, acknowledging, experiencing, understanding, and accepting the pieces of your life that were suppressed and fitting them into the spaces where they belong.

It is my opinion and experience that if you have been "working on yourself" to overcome a trauma for more than five years and you are having similar conversations in your fifth year that you were in the first year, then it's time to try a different strategy. If you would like to see a video of me teaching the flow chart in Figure 37, make sure to go to www.healthtovitality.com/videos to access the videos that accompany the book.

---

[40]   Maté Gabor (2019)
[41]   Maté Gabor (2017)

Integrating Emotional Communication

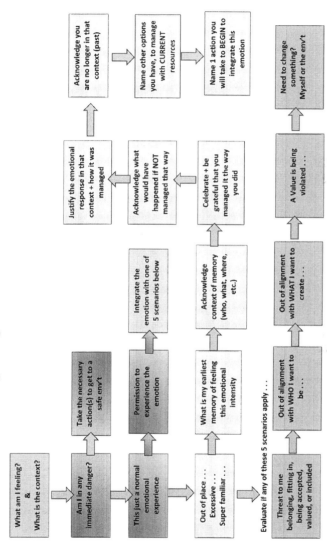

Fig 37: Emotional Integration Flow Chart from Matthew's ALIGN Course

CASE STUDY

"The Cozy Prison"

A gentleman named Mark came to see me for some help with his severe anxiety and sleeping troubles. He was a very successful physician, married with two beautiful daughters, and he lived in a beautiful home, minutes away from the beach. On paper, this guy had created the perfect life. As I got to know Mark better, I learned he was not really thrilled with his career. He said he felt very unfulfilled and had no real passion for what he did. He was a dermatologist and spent most of his days assessing different skin abnormalities and performing the same procedures over and over again. He found his days to be very tedious, mundane, and uninspiring. He was also very aware of the incredible things he had in his life which made his experience even worse. He would often share with me that he knew he should be grateful for all he had and that so many people in the world were not as fortunate as he was. This just led to additional feelings of guilt and shame.

At this point he had tried many different techniques to boost his lack of motivation and reduce his anxiety—some helped a little, but none were really getting him where he wanted to go. He wanted to feel inspired and passionate about life and was riddled with guilt and shame because he did not feel this way, knowing intellectually that he had so much that so many people lacked.

We dove into why he had chosen to be a doctor of dermatology, hoping to reignite his "why" and get him back on track. Turned out, this was something he never really wanted to do in the first place. He remembered when he was in his residency in medical school he kept thinking to himself, "I don't really want to be a doctor". I asked him why he went to medical school if he didn't want to be a doctor. He proceeded to tell me that as long as he could remember, his parents worried about the "unexpected" and always did their best to make sure they were prepared for the worst. He learned from a very young age to take the safe and secure routes, to not risk too much, and most importantly, to do what would keep himself and his family safe and secure.

To say he hit a home run on fulfilling this outcome would be an understatement—he nailed it! He had created an enormous amount of financial security and stability in his life. His family lacked nothing and had more than they could ever need. The only problem was that he felt empty inside, and on top of the emptiness he felt a ton of guilt for feeling that way. Every fiber of his being was screaming inside because something was seriously out of alignment. He wasn't living *his* life, he was living someone else's life—his parents' life. When you are living someone else's life script and not your own, you will experience feeling unfulfilled, empty, and dead inside.

This was an example of the adapted self designing and creating his whole life. And because that part of Mark was so successful in creating this life, his authentic self was left behind, leaving him feeling empty and unfulfilled. His adapted self had created a prison for his authentic self. Helping Mark get back in touch with his authentic self was the Big Rock we needed to address.

I have found this to be the most challenging space for people to navigate and change because they have made their lifestyle (and their loved ones) very cozy. The decision Mark and many others in this situation face is to either opt-in for temporary pain while transitioning lifestyles or opt-in for the long-term suffering of maintaining the prison of their status quo. When the current situation is painful, the motivation to take action to make a change is much easier to find. The only way someone ever decides to take action to make a change in their life is when the pain of staying where they are is greater than the perceived pain of changing. It is more difficult to take that action when the prison that holds our suffering is cozy. It becomes much more challenging to get to the turning point.

When someone is in this situation, the key is to make the idea of staying in the cozy prison more painful than the perceived pain or discomfort of leaving the prison. It is important to understand that there is a price for everything. There was a price for Mark to stay in his cozy prison and there was a price for him to leave it. Unfortunately, because of the coziness of the situation, the level of pain necessary to change direction needed to be amplified significantly.

One of the best ways to create enough pain inside of a cozy prison is to leverage potential future pain and start feeling it now. One of the exercises I gave Mark was to ask himself what life would look like if he decided to stay inside his daily suffering, continued to not get adequate sleep, and continued going through the motions of life. What impact would that have on his health, what impact would that have on the relationship with his wife, and what impact would it have on his children? I asked him to consider what example it provided his daughters. Did he want his daughters living someone else's life or did he want them to live the lives they were designed to live? Did he want to see his daughters sign up to live for their families and put all their needs aside because it was safer? Did he want to see them subjugating themselves to their husbands? I was intentionally being very specific and graphic to conjure up the pain that would be endured if changes were not made.

The good news for Mark is that these images conjured up enough future pain that he started taking some action to move in another direction. He got in touch with some of the things he was always passionate about and always wanted to do. One of these things was creating sports and outdoor activity camps for kids. Anytime he talked about being with his two daughters at their various sporting activities, he lit up. And every time he got back from a skiing trip or some outdoor activity with his girls, he was alive. It was clear this needed to be more integrated into his life going forward.

Mark and I are in the process of creating a transition out of his practice in the next five years and positioning himself to start different sport and activity summer camps for kids. It has been incredible to see life back in Mark's eyes.

Lean into Stress

If we don't want to mitigate, avoid, or manage stress, what do we want to do with it? We want to align with it. In Alia Crum's presentation "Gladstone Rethinks Stress with Mindset Expert Alia Crum"[42] and Kelly McGonigal's TedX talk[43], "How to Make Stress Your Friend", it is clearly shown that we need to completely redefine how we relate to stress. These two presentations illustrate the two sides of the stress coin or the paradox of stress. (Fig 38)

---

[42] Gladstone Institutes (2016)
[43] TED Talks (2013)

The Stress Paradox

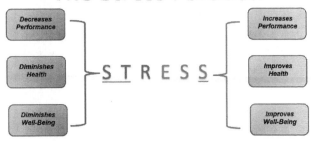

Fig 38: The Stress Paradox

On one side, there are countless studies on the negative impact of stress. One of the most recent studies done in 2017 connected emotional stress with cardiovascular disease.[44] I'm sure you don't need more studies to come up with examples of how stress can hinder your own performance and overall well-being. We have all personally experienced or witnessed someone underperforming in their job or role because they are too stressed. This is more commonly referred to as burn out. We have also seen stress do a number on our health and mental well-being.

On the flip side, stress has also been shown to increase performance by up-leveling our senses and speeding up our mental processing. We are familiar with examples of individuals who perform at peak levels when under stress. One of the best examples of this manifests when we have a deadline that is important to us. In these cases, the stress response kicks in but actually makes us sharper, more resilient, and gives us more energy. Performance is enhanced which has a positive impact on our well-being, making us more confident, tough, and resilient. It has also been shown that

---

[44] Takakol Ahmed and Ishai Amorina (2017)

our immunity is boosted during the stress response, making us more resistant to getting sick. If you think about the last time you were stressed out and driving hard toward resolving something or pursuing something, it is very unlikely that you got sick during the time of resolution or pursuit. As a matter of fact, you may have been able to operate at an abnormally high level with less sleep and minimal self-care. This is the superpower the stress response provides. The aftermath may have been a crash, but that is a result of turning off the stress response.

I experienced this first hand after I left the personal development organization in October of 2021. Leaving the organization meant that over 90 percent of my current income would disappear. Not only did I have a family to take care of but I was in the process of closing escrow on a home. To say it was a little stressful is an understatement.

The upside was after leaving this organization I got back in touch with what was really meaningful to me and the mission I had been on since the late 90s—exploring this new paradigm of vitality. I felt reborn, completely invigorated, and totally inspired.

Within the next two months, a colleague and I developed and launched a new set of personal development courses and started a new business together called Arena Method based on the famous Teddy Roosevelt quote, "Man in the Arena." We were determined to create a program that aligned people's mindset with their innate biology. Our passion and excitement as we created a personal development system that empowered individuals to create what they wanted without being dependent on the system, was through the roof. We worked eighteen hour days for a month and loved every single second of it.

What made this possible was that my stress response was fully activated. It was the reason we could produce what we produced in such a short period of time. People in our courses were convinced we worked on these courses for years, but we created all of it in less than two months. Not only did I create the Arena Method courses, but I also wrote and published this book within the first year of leaving the organization. This is a case where the stress response was essential to up-leveling performance, focus, and determination to make these things happen.

This begs the question, which one is it? Is stress good or bad? Does it kill us or make us stronger? And how do we get the benefits of the stress response without the negative effects? The good news is there is a clear and proven answer to these questions. First off, stress is neither good nor bad, just like electricity isn't good or bad. Electricity can be used to light up the world or electrocute you. Stress is no different. Like most things, it all depends on how it's used and applied. The latest research has shown that the determining factor as to whether stress has a positive or a negative impact is dependent solely on one's mindset toward stress. If stress is looked at as a bad thing, and therefore the focus is to avoid, manage, or mitigate it, the effects of stress will be harmful. However, if stress is looked at as an asset, something that the body is doing to support you, and that you can leverage, the negative effects are limited—and in many cases eliminated completely.

The work of researchers like Alia Crum of Stanford and others have developed what is now known as the stress mindset theory:

> "Stress mindset theory suggests that positive
> stress beliefs lead to positive, rather than negative,
> outcomes when engaging with stressors."[45]

---

[45] Kilby C and Sherman K (2016)

If we assume the body is on our side and isn't doing something to kill us, ruin our day, or inconvenience us, we may be able to see the stress response in a different way. When the stress response is activated, the body increases heart rate, increases respiration, raises our body temperature, and increases our blood pressure. Why would it do this? What is it doing?

All of these actions are doing one very specific thing, they are mobilizing resources to take action. Our biology is in high action to support us in addressing whatever situation that has surfaced that we *care* about. It has our back! Not only does it secrete powerful neuro-hormones like adrenaline to spring into action, but it also secretes a hormone called oxytocin. Oxytocin is a fascinating hormone that has gotten a lot of attention lately. In some circles it is referred to as the "cuddle" hormone because it increases the drive for connection and closeness to others. Now why would our physiology release the cuddle hormone with the stress response? Could it be because when we are facing a situation we care about, reaching out to others for support would be useful? It not only provides more resources to us in our time of need, but it also biologically nudges us to connect and seek support from others. Wow, the body is amazing! It has thought of everything!

One thing that has proven time and time again to diminish the negative impact of stressful effects and trauma for individuals is connection—the connection of supporting others and allowing others to support us. The unfortunate reality is so many people are not only trying to numb the stress response with different modalities and techniques but are also white knuckling themselves through stressful events with narratives like, "I can do this myself," "I don't need any help," and "I should be able to handle this." These narratives and strategies put us in direct conflict with our biological processes.

I experienced this when I was managing the team of practitioners who worked for me at my clinic in Los Angeles.

In my stressful states, I never reached out for help, never asked anyone for support, and always held it in—relying only on myself to get things done. This was the kiss of death for me and my team. What it created was a lack of connection and communication with them all. I continued to muscle my way through getting everything done, which meant nothing got done to any high standards. This created a lot of uncertainty and anxiety amongst the team, and most of them eventually left to do their own thing. As they each left, I blamed them for betraying me and was very angry and disappointed with them. Looking back on this today, I completely understand why they left. I did not fulfill my job as a leader and did not work with them to create a cohesive unit where we all trusted and communicated with each other to fulfill a common goal. I am grateful for this lesson because I am now able to coach and support business and leadership teams to not make the same mistakes and encourage them to create strong coherent leadership teams who can trust each other.

So how do we position ourselves to align our stress response in an advantageous way? There is a very simple process that can be used to help align yourself with the body's stress response and it is very similar to how we partner with our emotions.

Step One: Position Your Mindset

> Assume the stress response is happening on your behalf and that it is not a hindrance or a sign of weakness.

Step Two: Name the Stress

> Naming the stress means naming the emotion you are feeling and distinguishing the feeling from what is happening. This is important because it directs the

brain activity from the brainstem to the neocortex which allows us to access rational thinking and problem solving.

"I'm feeling _____."

Step Three: Acknowledge Why

It is important to acknowledge *WHY* you are stressed and welcome it. This can be done with a simple sentence:

"I'm feeling _____ because I care about _____."

Reminding yourself that the stress is there because you *care* about something takes away the negative aspect of the stress response. And naming why you are stressed gives your brain something to focus on to begin directing the resources to solve whatever threat or situation needs attention.

NOTE: If you want to become dissociated and detached from your emotions then train yourself never to ask why you feel something.

Step Four: Outcome and Action

Identify the ultimate outcome that would resolve the situation or problem that you are facing..

Below is an example that I have walked clients through that many of us can relate to—losing your job. This is an event that will most likely activate our stress response.

Step One: Position Your Mindset

> As our heart rate increases, our palms get sweaty, and our blood pressure rises, it is important to acknowledge that the body is jumping into action to provide the resources to address the fact that we will need to be in high action to deal with the situation.

Step Two: Name the Stress

> Acknowledge the emotions you were experiencing when you found out you lost your job—emotions like fear, anxiety, and possibly overwhelm. You can acknowledge them with a simple statement, "I'm feeling anxious."

Step Three: Acknowledge Why

"I feel anxious about losing my job because I care about taking care of my family."

Step Four: Outcome and Action

> Outcome could be to provide for your family. This is an outcome we can directly control or influence by getting a new job. We would want to channel the resources the body is providing us to start tuning up our resumes, sending them out, and going on interviews.

Relating to the stress response as a friend and not a foe positions you to take advantage and leverage the powerful resources your physiology provides you. It allows you to partner with your biology to solve problems that arise in life and ensure that the most important and meaningful things you care about are taken care of. This is another topic I go over in my ALIGN course in greater depth.

CASE STUDY

"It's Time to Trust Yourself"

Jamie was a top sales executive in the technology industry. At every company she had worked for, she was consistently one of the top three performers. She was an incredibly sweet, caring, and sensitive individual, not someone whom you'd picture thriving in this type of environment. She was also wicked sharp and extremely good with people, always looking to create the best experience for her clients and over-delivering as much as she could.

It is important to note that Jamie had been involved in some personal development systems that had identified a pattern of self-doubt, insecurity, and anger—emotions she had been trying to shake for many years. This was an experience that she seemed to have time and time again, not only in her career, but in her romantic relationships. It was quite frustrating for her because she was working so hard on herself to fix what she had been told were "destructive ways of being". Historically, she struggled to create healthy boundaries with boyfriends, colleagues, and superiors at work. Jamie also engaged in many destructive habits like binging and purging as well as drinking to the point of complete inebriation.

Jamie specifically came to me for some guidance with a situation at one of her jobs. She had been recruited by a company and was promised certain opportunities and positions by them. However, when she transferred there, they didn't follow through on any of their promises. She was infinitely frustrated, felt betrayed, and fell into a hole of self-doubt and insecurity.

She told me she was really angry because she felt she was lied to. She noticed that the self-doubt and insecurity had begun to dominate her experience at work. She told me this was her pattern, and she didn't know how to overcome it. She had tried all the techniques of accepting the emotions and breathing through them until they passed. Although it seemed to take the edge off at times, they continued to return over and over again.

She explained that she had these destructive patterns because of some childhood experiences and was convinced she was broken and no matter what she did, the ghosts from her past would always haunt her.

That was it! The Big Rock. She didn't trust her emotional communication because she was told that her emotional communication system was her problem. All she was doing was trying to get those feelings of self-doubt, anger, and insecurity to go away. I knew what I had to do—teach her how to listen and integrate these emotions so they would no longer haunt her.

I shared with her that feeling these emotions was not an indication that she was broken, flawed, or reliving something from her past. I invited her to consider that these feelings were actually attempting to communicate something very important and were there because they were supporting her—not trying to sabotage her.

We considered that the emotion of anger was a communication that one of her core values was being violated and it was a signal to pay attention. The insecurity and self-doubt could be spot-on in their communication that this is not a place where she can be successful and still live in alignment with the experience of life she most valued. To be successful in this environment, she would have to put those needs aside and tolerate being treated in ways that were not in alignment with the culture and relationships she yearned to have in her life. The environments she was exposed to in her career were very disrespectful to women and didn't hold the values she held as important like integrity, kindness, and honesty. They tended to be more cutthroat and manipulative.

Because she was told that these emotions were destructive patterns from her past, she never trusted them and never considered they were actually there to help her and that she wasn't broken at all! Her journey was about learning to trust herself again and assume that what she was feeling wasn't a misfiring of her biology, but it was actually her biology doing an exceptional job. It was letting her know that she, and her environment, were not aligned with the life that was most important for her to live.

Jamie was able to navigate out of those technology sales jobs and by continuing to trust herself and her intuition she is now following her dream of starting her own business. She is also currently in one of the most healthy romantic relationships in her life.

Trilogy of Vitality Pillar III Mindset Summary

➤ Pursue meaning and purpose not "positive emotions" like happiness

➤ Emotions are part of your powerful communication system, not something to pursue or eliminate.

➤ Align your emotional communication system to direct you towards what is most meaningful to you

➤ Embrace the stress response as an ally, not as something that you need to avoid, manage, or eliminate

TRILOGY OF VITALITY

PUTTING IT ALL TOGETHER

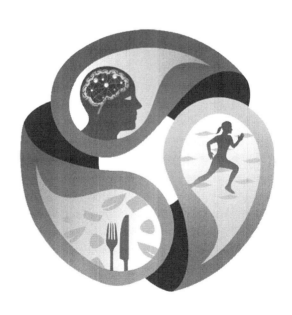

Chapter 8

IT'S NEVER TOO LATE

The beautiful thing about our body and brain is their ability to adapt. The brain's ability to learn, grow, evolve and adapt is called neuroplasticity and is by far one of our biggest assets as humans. Although the plasticity of the brain, its ability to learn, is the greatest before the age of twenty-five, our brain always has the ability to change, evolve, and grow. The best way to leverage this powerful trait, is to put ourselves in environments that align with who we want to be and what we want to learn.

I'm going to share with you three principles and a framework that I have found to provide a context and tools that has given people the ability create the best internal and external environment to grow, learn, and evolve, in the most optimal way. They will also empower you in any situation you may find yourself in, will support you in managing any conflict in your life, and leverage the unexpected events that occur to accelerate progress. The clients who have learned and implemented these vitality principles and vitality framework, range in age from thirteen to ninety years old. You will read about one of these clients at the end of this chapter who fulfilled her lifelong dream at the age of eighty-eight! Let's begin.

The Vitality Principles

1. Ownership
2. Growth Mindset
3. Twelve-Week Chunks

Vitality Principle #1: Ownership

Julian B. Rotter, a psychologist in the 1950s, created a theoretical construct on how individuals perceive their reality. He called it the locus of control[46]. Locus of control is the degree to which individuals believe that they are in control of their lives. He identified two perceptions, internal locus of control and external locus of control. Internal locus of control was when an individual was focused on their own ability, what they had control over, and their belief that their effort made a difference. External locus of control was focused more on the external environment dictating their life experience, the things they didn't have control over, and their lack of efficacy. External locus of control can also be thought of as a victim mindset—you are a victim of your circumstances and there is nothing you can do about it.

There are certainly things over which we have absolutely no control and it is important to identify what those things are, but it is far more important to identify what you can control. I have never met an individual or heard of any circumstances where someone had control over *nothing*. Even in the most extreme situations, an internal locus of control is applicable and extremely powerful. Just ask Mahatma Gandhi, Viktor Frankl and Nelson Mandela.

---

[46] Wikipedia. "Locus of Control" (2022)

Whenever I am working with a couple or an individual who is struggling in a relationship, the first thing I have them look at is the influence they have had on the relationship. It is common when I first meet these individuals for them to tell me all the things that are wrong with their partner, child, boss, or whomever. They want me to help them manage, deal with or fix this other person. This is a great example of an external locus of control. They are primarily focused on the other person as the problem in the relationship. As you may have heard, it takes two to tango—it is *never* one person; it is always both. There is always something that can be done, if we own our part in it. From there, we have extraordinary power to influence a positive change.

Owning what you can control is essential to navigating any situation in life and is critical in situations where there is conflict. Think of what you can control as the immediate space around you, which includes yourself. I refer to it as the sphere of ownership. When things get complicated, make your world small and focus there. Imagine a three-foot space all around you and start assessing and taking action in that sphere.

Things that are in the sphere of ownership are:

1. How you think about something
2. Your actions

Owning how you think about or perceive something and the actions you take are *all* in your control. This makes you completely responsible and accountable for their impact. This is ownership and what creates the empowerment to take control and move forward.

These principles have saved Eve and me on multiple occasions. Most recently we used these principles to manage a challenging situation with our residence. We had moved into our current house as renters in November of 2019. We had been stashing money away for a few years so we would be in a position to purchase a house in 2023. When we moved into the house, we asked the owners if they had any plans to sell the house in the future and that if they did, we would be very interested in purchasing it from them. The house was exactly what we had envisioned owning. The owners told us they were planning on selling it in 2023 because that was when they would need the capital for their son's college education. It was perfect!

Fast forward a few months later, we entered 2020 and we all know what happened that year—global pandemic. By mid-March, the whole country had shut down and nobody knew what this would mean or how long the pandemic would last. Fortunately for me, my business continued to thrive as I was able to transition all my offerings to virtual presentations. As the year progressed, things continued to stay shut down and in September of that year (2020), we received a call from the owners. They told us that due to unexpected circumstances, they were going to need to sell the house "now". They even offered it to us at about $50,000 dollars less than current market value. It was exactly what we had dreamed of, but, unfortunately, we were in no position to buy it at that time. We were really upset - we had not even been in the house for a year and now we would have to move again, and lose an incredible opportunity.

I went into a brief tailspin, feeling super frustrated and overwhelmed by the whole situation. Then Eve chimed in and said, "Matt, don't you teach people to focus on what they do have control over and take action from there?" The timing of that reminder couldn't have been better. We sat down and used our energy to brainstorm our options. We decided our first option would be to ask the owners if they could give us a little more time to get our finances together so we would be able to purchase the home. I would need to call in a few favors and borrow some money, but I thought I'd be able to pull it off if they gave us an extra six months. We asked them if they would be willing to sell it to us at the end of the first quarter in 2021. The response we received back was music to our ears. The owners not only said they would be able to do that, they said they could give us until the *end* of 2021 to get our finances together! In addition they repeated their offer to sell the house at a price that was approximately $50,000 less than the market value at that time. We were floored and very, very grateful. They asked for a good faith deposit of about $20,000. We could apply it to the purchase of the house but would not be refundable if we ended up being unable to purchase the home. They also made it very clear that if the market crashed, we would still be on the hook to purchase it at the negotiated price. On the flip side, if the market skyrocketed, we could be getting a great deal.

We went into immediate action and created a strategy that we were able to execute over the next year to get our finances in the best shape they had ever been in, with the highest credit score we've ever had, and with enough cash to be able to purchase the house in October of 2021. At the time we actually purchased the home, the value of the property had almost doubled. If we hadn't leveraged the stress of that situation, taken extreme ownership, and focused on our sphere of influence, we would never have been able to buy it.

One of the most impactful places where the sphere of ownership can be leveraged is in relationships. In the case study below, I supported a young woman to help keep her marriage together and avoid what seemed like an inevitable divorce.

CASE STUDY

"We just aren't meant to be together."

A young lady named Lauren came to me looking for some support for her marriage. She was in her late thirties and had two children. Her primary complaint was that she and her husband were simply too different. She wanted to talk about her life, aspirations, and goals and he didn't. She also felt like he was apathetic about life which made it very difficult for them to connect. Lauren told me that she had been thinking about these things for years. To some degree, she kind of knew from the beginning of the relationship that they weren't "meant to be."

This is where the tip of the Big Rock started to appear. When she described all this to me, I said that it sounded like *she* was never committed to this relationship from day one. I then told her that I believed, because she was never committed, the relationship had never had a chance and I wasn't surprised that she was where she was. That definitely got her attention and she began defending her position. She said she had given it a chance to work for years, but he just couldn't give her what she needed or wanted. She also mentioned that because she had been trying to make it work for so long, now it was time to put herself first and do what she wanted. I then asked her how she had been trying to make it work. She gave me examples of the chances she had given her husband to step up and meet her needs but now she was done.

This was the rest of the Big Rock. She took zero ownership for the role she played in the current state of her relationship. I needed to help her take ownership and step into an internal locus of control so she could actually influence the relationship in a way that could save it. I next asked her what she wanted in a relationship— what experiences, activities, interactions, and so on, was she looking for? She mentioned she wanted someone who loved her unconditionally, accepted her for who she was, and valued her for everything she does. I then asked her a very simple question that stopped her dead in her tracks. I asked her if she was offering that to her husband? Or was she waiting for him to do it so she felt safe enough to do it herself? This led us down another path where she mentioned she was afraid to share herself with him because it would hurt too much if he didn't reciprocate. She recounted some past experiences where she had opened her heart to someone and gotten severely burned.

I shared with her my rule for relationships, "Go first." I find in many of these types of relationships there are two individuals, each waiting for the other person to make it alright and safe enough to open up their hearts and connect. Owning one's side of the relationship and going all in by being vulnerable and opening your heart is the only chance anyone has to create the kind of intimate partnership we desire. The inherent risk is that it is absolutely possible they will not reciprocate and yes, it will sting. It's supposed to sting, and at times it will be painful. But it is through these moments that you will learn to align your expectations realistically and know how to evaluate the capacity other people have to meet these expectations.

There is no way to avoid painful experiences in life, but we can avoid the suffering. Pain is something to leverage, it is a communication that allows us to make a calibration. Suffering is what happens when we try to avoid pain. It would be like having a tooth ache but not going to the dentist because you fear the pain of fixing the tooth. Instead, you suffer with the discomfort of a decaying tooth longer than necessary. Many people opt out of temporary pain to suffer forever. In my Relationships Course, I go into much more depth about the methods that can be used to discern and implement many different strategies to connect. You can learn more about that course at www.healthtovitality.com/Relationships

When you live your life with an open heart, there will be times when it will be painful. However, it is possible for you to learn how to use discernment to engage with an open heart and manage the expectations in a relationship in a way that will minimize the painful events. Although you cannot eliminate all of the painful situations, you can certainly make them the exception over time and live the majority of your life creating the deeply connected relationships that you want.

I have opened my heart and trusted some mentors to have my best interests in mind when guiding me in my life's decisions. To find out that guidance was being used and manipulated to serve their best interests -and not mine - was very painful. Coming to terms with this sense of betrayal stung a lot, and I felt like a complete fool. In those moments, there was no part of me who wanted to trust anyone ever again. Once I learned this principle of ownership, I was able to apply it to own my side of the relationship and how I influenced the outcome. I looked back at those situations and evaluated what role I had played and what I could learn from the experience. I saw signs I had missed and moments when I didn't trust my own intuitive and emotional communication systems - and I should have. As a result, today I'm able to continue to open my heart to my current and new relationships, with much more ability to navigate boundaries and communications within them. This was the opportunity Lauren had with her husband.

Lauren began taking small steps toward opening her heart to her husband, things like sitting next to him when he sat on the couch watching sports—an activity that had previously driven her crazy because she felt he was ignoring her. I suggested she just go sit next to him, place her hand on his knee, and smile at him. When she did this, after his initial shock, he grabbed the remote, turned off the TV and started talking to her.

Little things like this add up over time and create the space for incredibly connected relationships. From that day forward, Lauren continued to "go first." They are still married and continue nurturing their connection each day.

Taking "Extreme Ownership", to borrow a concept from X-Navy Seal and author, Jocko WIllink, is the absolute first step in positioning yourself to access a life of vitality. From this place you are now in a position to learn everything you need to know and to create the life you deserve to live. This is where principle #2 comes in.

Vitality Principle #2: Growth Mindset

The second vitality principle is aligning yourself with a growth mindset. This sets the stage for you to embrace learning - something you are designed to do until your last breath. Growth mindset was a concept created by American psychologist Carol Dweck. According to Dweck's research, some individuals believed their success in life was based on their innate ability (fixed mindset), while others believed success was determined by hard work, learning, training, and perseverance (growth mindset). She showed that individuals with a fixed mindset had a significant antagonistic attitude toward failure since they felt it was a direct attack on their innate ability or identity, while individuals who had a growth mindset didn't mind or fear failure because they looked at it as an opportunity to grow, learn, and evolve.

"In a fixed mindset students believe their basic abilities, their intelligence, their talents, are just fixed traits. They have a certain amount and that's that, and then their goal becomes to look smart all the time and never look dumb. In a growth mindset students understand that their talents and abilities can be developed through effort, good teaching and persistence. They don't necessarily think everyone's the same or anyone can be Einstein, but they believe everyone can get smarter if they work at it."[47]

A growth mindset also aligns us with our biological processes of motivation, purpose, and meaning. Motivation is a drive that is hardwired into our biological processes and is directed by one molecule, dopamine. The amount of dopamine that is in supply at any moment in your body will determine how motivated you are. The key thing to understand about dopamine is that it is more actively secreted when we are in pursuit of something, not when we arrive at the reward. The growth mindset is effective because it keeps our baseline dopamine level high; this equates to motivation that is sustained by embracing the effort, the journey, and the growth rather than the reward at the end of the journey.

Someone with a growth mindset looks at obstacles as opportunities to grow, rewards the effort much more than the accomplishment, is open minded, and is always pursuing growth and learning. All of this aligns us with our biological wiring.

That being said, it is important to understand that nobody lives primarily in one mindset over the other. We all have areas in our life where we orient more with a growth

---

[47]   Dweck Carol (2012)

mindset and others that are more fixed. We may look at a skill or activity that we enjoy with a growth mindset and are excited to learn the nuances of that skill and celebrate the learning process. We also have areas that we may orient to with a fixed mindset and relate to something as, "well, I'm just not good at that." I would bet that the places in your life where you find more meaning and fulfillment are the ones where you bring a growth mindset.

I have found that orienting to this mindset is essential for achieving a meaningful and purposeful life. Growth mindset has you lean into the challenges and leverage them to help you reach your goals. On the other hand, having a fixed mindset and going through life avoiding challenges, taking the easy road, and settling, limits you to a life that is much less than it could be. When pursuing what is most meaningful to you, it isn't a matter of if there will be challenges, it is just a matter of when. Living the life you are here to live will be hard at times, and sometimes may seem impossible—but it will always be worth pursuing.

In the case study with Lauren, from the fixed mindset, her relationship was doomed and hopeless. Because she was brave enough to evolve to a growth mindset and lean into the challenges she was facing with her husband, there was a chance of them repairing and expanding their relationship for the better. In many of the situations she faced, it wasn't easy for Lauren to do what she did. At first she went kicking and screaming, but she stayed the course. Once again I commend her on her courage and resolve to lean in and do it anyway. I can tell you she would absolutely say, "It was worth it."

Vitality Principles #3: 12-Week Chunk Principle

This final principle is the strategy to which I attribute some of my greatest accomplishments. It is living life twelve weeks at a time. I have been able to create an entire business, write this book, eliminate debt, and double my net worth using this principle. There are three main reasons why this is an important principle and strategy to implement.

1. Laser-like focus
2. Confident commitments
3. Makes time matter

The first thing that 12-Week Chunking creates is a *laser-like focus*. It shrinks your world to a twelve-week period of time which allows you to hone in on specific goals at a very high level. Focusing on what you want to accomplish and what you need to do on a weekly and daily basis for twelve weeks is much easier to manage than orienting to longer-term goals like 1, 3, 5, or 20-year periods. There is a place for bigger-picture thinking, but it is important to shrink most things down to an intermediate range that you can lock in on.

The second reason why the 12-Week Chunking is beneficial is that it allows you to confidently make binding commitments; it is a relatively short period of time which makes it easier to follow through. Committing to something for many years, or even one year, is a little more risky because you don't know what you don't know. When starting a new journey, I find that it is better to take it slow and keep your eyes open. This can happen to people in relationships who get off to a hot start. It can be easy to get wrapped up in the famous "honeymoon phase" and make long-term commitments. Most of the time, people don't even realize what they just signed up for and often regret it down the road.

The other place where I see 12 Week Chunking have value is in coaching younger professionals, especially right out of college. So many have the idea that they need to know what they should do as a career for the rest of their life. This is insane. Although there are some individuals who have known what they wanted to do as a career their whole life, I have found this to be the exception. I often advise individuals who are unsure of what direction to go, to make a shorter commitment to things. Commit to something for a year, six months, or even ninety days when applicable. It is necessary to experience life to figure out that you don't know what you don't know. Over time we grow, evolve, and gain experiential knowledge and operational intelligence. Making long-term commitments from a place of ignorance often leads to regret. What makes sense to commit to now, may not make sense a year from now.

Commitment is an essential part of fulfilling any outcome, but making sure to not overcommit or commit too far into the future, especially when you can't see that far, is an important thing to be mindful of. When you decide to focus on what is most important to fulfill and do in the next twelve weeks, it is much easier to manage. The other thing this cultivates is the ability to trust in what you commit to. If you consistently make short-term commitments and fulfill them, you will trust that you are a person who fulfills commitments.

The third reason the 12 Week Chunk Principle is effective is because it makes time matter more. This is probably the most important of the three. Too often, we put off what we could accomplish today because we tell ourselves, "I have time." We don't realize the precious value of every moment of every day. Every day you live is a day you cannot live again. Looking at your life in a 12-week period of time, and orienting to those 12 weeks as the only thing that exists, puts you in a mindset where you realize that every moment of every day counts.

I used this twelve-week chunking strategy to write this book. When I met with my writing coach the first time and told him what my intentions were in writing this book, he told me the most important step is getting the rough draft done. He also shared with me that 80 percent of the people who say they want to write a book never finish their rough draft. That is all I needed to hear—that wasn't going to be me! I pulled out my planner and designed what I was going to commit to for the next twelve weeks to get my rough draft completed. I wasn't exactly sure how many words this book was going to be, but I was told nonfiction books are around 40–60,000 words, so I used 50,000 words as my guideline. To write 50,000 words in twelve weeks meant I had to write about 4,000 words a week. I looked at my calendar and saw that I could easily commit to writing four days a week for about 60–90 minutes each time. The goal and commitment became very clear: write 1,000 words four times a week for twelve straight weeks. I continued with these twelve-week commitments to complete the book and get it published in less than one year. I met individuals over the past year in different writers' circles who have been trying to write their book for the last five years!

The Habits Course that I designed walks you step by step through naming what is most important to you in your life now and honing in on a specific goal to fulfill in 12 weeks. People who have taken this course have accomplished more in 12 weeks than most people accomplish in an entire year. Go to www.healthtovitality.com/Habits for more details.

The Players of Vitality

The vitality principles of ownership, growth mindset, and twelve-week chunking set you up with a solid strategy to engage in the game of life. But as in any game, it is important for you to understand the players. Knowing the players gives you more clarity on what is in your sphere of ownership. This gives you the ability to own what is yours to own and influence the areas where you do not have direct control. When I create an intention to manifest something in my life, I consider and acknowledge these three players because I believe they will be involved in making it happen. Aligning and working with these players has been the key to creating the life I know today. These three players are:

1. Our Essence
2. Our Vehicle
3. The Environment

Our Essence

When you look at human history throughout time in every part of the world there has been a consistent orientation to a world that exists beyond the mortal or material plane. The representations of this orientation can be seen as far back as the Bhagavad-Gita, which was written over 5000 years ago, the Muses of Homer's "Iliad" published about 762 BCE, Lao Tsu's Tao Te Ching (China) from about the fifth century BCE, the Jewish/Christian scriptures and Islam's Koran, continuing throughout history to some of the most recent work of Dr. Joe Dispenza, in what he refers to as the "quantum realm". These are all examples of humans trying to explain the unknown. Having answers for things we can't explain is a way that humans have been regulating themselves from the beginning of civilization. I have found that these frameworks can be very supportive and can also be very destructive. It is helpful when these explanations create a framework that teaches us to respect each other and our planet, uniting us as a coherent community. It is very destructive when it pins "my god/s" against "your god/s" or claims that if you don't believe what it teaches, you are "doomed". One trend that has been happening repeatedly throughout human existence is that the advancements of science consistently shrink the unknown world. It turns out that the lightning and thunder you hear during storms is not Thor riding his chariot across the sky smashing his hammer on the earth or an enemy. I share all this with you to create some context for what I am going to say regarding our human essence. It is simply a framework that some day may be explained by science more thoroughly. I use it as a framework because I have found that it allows me to access my greatest potential and unites me with humanity and our planet.

The foundational idea behind this essence framework is rooted in an idea that has also been around for tens of thousands of years. It is the idea that there is a presence, an energy, an intelligence, a "consciousness", that is present in all things and unites all things in the universe. And yes, it can be as simple as "the force", for you Star Wars fans. This idea is where the idea of our essence originates.

There have been many words used to describe this presence, whether it is being referenced as a global presence or a presence that inhabits each individual. Words like soul, god, life force, chi, shakti, consciousness, presence, energy, and countless others. The greater or more global presence is often referred to as a higher consciousness, intelligence, or a divine being. Words like soul or life force are often references to what inhabits an individual. The connection and interplay of these ideas, is what an artist will refer to when they share their source of inspiration, "It just came to me". Salvador Dali famously saw images in his dreams that had a major influence on his paintings. I believe this is all the work of this presence and our essence is the aspect of this presence that is always interacting and communicating with this higher, more global consciousness. Learning how to connect to our unique essence and interact with the greater consciousness, is a framework that I and many others have found to be extremely powerful.

There are three ways I have found to leverage and use our essence and its connection with this greater intelligence, to live the most extraordinary lives. They are the three essential roles, I believe our essence plays:

1.   Identifying our mission and purpose
2.   Access to our intuition
3.   Uniting us with humankind and the universe

Mission and Purpose

I believe it is our essence that makes each of us unique. My belief is that we have all come into human incarnation to offer our unique expression of consciousness to the world at this time. Just like there are no two fingerprints that are the same, I do not believe there are two signatures of consciousness that are the same. Every human being on the planet has an expression of consciousness that only exists within that individual. It is in this vibration and frequency that our mission and purpose live. This expression of essence is most evident when we are young children. It can be seen in every child—that wonder for the world and interest in exploring and knowing everything. It expresses within each child in unique ways as evidenced by each child's natural affinity—their interests, demeanor, and temperament. Although it is strongest when we are children, it is present and communicating to us throughout our lives.

One of the more common ways this is referenced in many personal development fields is your "why". Simon Sinek really emphasized the importance of your *why* when he delivered his famous Ted Talk.[48] Our *why* is essentially our purpose and mission. It is what makes life worth living. It is the thing to which we tie the most value and importance. It is the thing we get the most resilience and strength from to overcome and persevere through life's greatest challenges. It is when we are in touch and aligned with this *why*, and connected to this string of consciousness that lives inside of us, that we feel most complete, whole, and fulfilled.

One thing that is important to mention is that a mission and purpose doesn't have to be some grandiose plan that is going to change the world on a global, international, or national scale. It can and most likely is going to have a significant and essential impact on your immediate world— your relationships, family, and communities.

One of the things I encourage my clients to assume is that whatever has happened or is happening to you now, is and always has been, somehow aligned with your purpose. It may not always make sense at the time, but I have found, both for myself and countless clients, that this orientation positions you to see the alignment. More importantly, it allows you to leverage whatever has happened, or is happening, to move you forward and propel you toward your *why*.

This is exactly the perspective Eve reminded me of when we received the call from our landlords about their need to sell the house. She encouraged me to take a step back

---

[48] Sinek Simon (2020)

and focus on what we can control, and she pointed out that maybe this was happening for a reason we could not see at the moment. If we assumed it was happening *for* us and not *to* us, we could see how to align what was happening with what we ultimately wanted to create. This perspective was exactly what enabled us to purchase the house a year later at a 50 percent discount.

To get to this perspective, it is important to create space to take a step back. I call this getting to 20,000 feet. My first mentor, Lenny Parracino, shared an analogy with me when he was teaching me how to evaluate human motion. He told me you have to be like a Black Hawk helicopter when you are doing the assessment. A Black Hawk helicopter is a military helicopter used to fly above a combat zone, survey the area from above, descend into the areas needing support, and get back out quickly so it isn't shot down. This is a perfect analogy for life as well. Any time things are complicated, I am reminded of the Black Hawk helicopter and how I need to get out of the minutiae of what is happening, and get to 20,000 feet where I can see a different perspective.

It is also important to elevate to 50,000 thousand feet at times to get an even bigger perspective on things. This is when I am able to see my life as a whole. It is from this perspective I can see the presence and work of my essence. When I reflect on my life and recall some of the toughest, most challenging events and periods in my life, I can see clearly how they served my present mission and purpose. And although some were excruciatingly painful, I can now see the capacity and ability I gained through those experiences and how they were essential to my ability to fulfill and pursue my mission.

The *AIM Course* that I developed is designed to get you in touch with your meaning and purpose. I walk you through a series of exercises that help you get in touch with your essence so you can tap into your purpose. From there I help you identify what the most impactful next step would be for you to take, regardless of where you may be. I then help you put together a simple but powerful action plan so you can move forward with clarity and confidence.

Intuition

The second role our essence plays is being the access point to our intuition. Intuition is the knowledge that exists beyond our intellect. It is the knowledge we have without any reason or evidence. The HeartMath Institute has done some incredible research on intuition. It has correlated the ability to access this incredible resource with the presence of certain physiological conditions in our body. These conditions are when the body is in a state of complete coherence, a state of quietness and clarity. HeartMath defines this state as "Heart Coherence". They have identified three types of intuition that can be accessed in this state: implicit knowledge, energetic sensitivity, and nonlocal.[49]

Implicit knowledge refers to the brain's ability to take in all of its experiences, learnings, and stimuli over time and begin to recognize patterns at a high rate which can translate to mastery. An example of this is a very experienced doctor or nurse who meets with a patient for a few minutes, immediately "knows" what is wrong with the patient, and takes immediate action that saves the patient's life. Another example of implicit knowledge is when you have an insight that helps you solve a problem you've been thinking about. This type of intuition is basically an example of our brain's capacity.

---

[49] HeartMath˚ Institute (2019)

The second type of intuition, energetic sensitivity, is our nervous system's ability to sense energetic signals in the environment and in other individuals and integrate the communication of those signals. An example of this is empathy or the sense that someone is staring at you.

The third type is nonlocal, which is a sense of foreknowledge. An example of this is when you have a sudden urge to reach out to someone you know, or check on a loved one you are not with only to find they needed you in that moment. This is very common with mothers and their children—it is famously referred to as mother's intuition. I believe this is the work of the presence that lives inside all of us. It is able to communicate with the essence that lives in all things. The HeartMath Institute has conducted studies that measured this nonlocal intuition. One of their most impactful studies was one that showed people's ability to accurately predict random pictures that were being shown on a computer screen. These pictures were ones that were consistently used to create intense emotional responses in people. What they found was that if a future event was emotionally relevant, their heart could produce a signal alerting them of the emotion that was associated with the picture, before the picture was shown or the event took place.

I believe the connection HeartMath has found between our hearts and intuition is not a coincidence. When we are connected and aligned with our hearts, we are most connected to our own essence, the essence of others, and our environment. Someday science will be able to measure and confirm the existence of this universal essence. Which brings me to the final significance of our essence.

Unity

When we are connected to and aligned with this infinite presence inside us, the common experience is the feeling of being connected to everyone and everything. When doing specific deep meditative practices for long periods of time, there is a state that is reached giving you an experience beyond the body. During these meditations, it is not unusual to feel connected and at one with other people and nature. There is a state of profound peace and wholeness that is experienced. When deeply entrenched in these experiences, things seem perfect and there is nothing you feel needs to be done. All ambitions are gone and the only thing that occurs to you is to just *be*.

You don't have to go into deep meditative practices to experience this. One of the places I have found where most people find this state of peace, connection, and wholeness is when they are in nature. Nature seems to give many people access to this experience of oneness.

I believe it is important to comment about individuals who strive to embody this state at all times. I have known individuals who engage in practices that intensely immerse them in this experience. It can be used and become a way to avoid difficult circumstances or completely disconnect themselves from reality. The result I've often seen from this is complete dissociation. In some spiritual practices and teachings, the goal is to actually live in this space - to become "unattached". You may have heard the saying, "attachment is the root of all suffering". Accomplishing this state of being "unattached" is seen to be the ultimate accomplishment. Commonly referred to as the state of enlightenment. But as we discussed in the previous chapter, the one way to eliminate stress ("suffering") is to eliminate caring - or to be "unattached". It seems to me that aspiring to live a life free of attachment is exactly the opposite of living a life of connection or vitality. I would recommend being extremely careful if you are making this your ultimate goal.

That being said, I do believe this experience is beneficial and connecting to this space is valuable when it is used to build coherence within ourselves and with humanity. I truly believe if we all spent a little more time connecting to this presence, we would feel more connected to each other as brothers and sisters in and from our own humanity. We would treat and respect our planet at a much higher level. There would be a lot less discrimination, fear, and hatred toward people who are different from us. If you would like a twenty-minute meditation that is designed to help you become more connected to your essence, go to www.healthtovitality. com/resources. Now that we have an understanding of the sacredness of our essence, let's explore where it lives.

The Vehicle

What allows our essence to explore the experience of being human is its access to a vehicle. The vehicle is the body. Like our essence, human life would not be possible without a body. The combination of the two gives us the ability to experience what it is to be human. The vehicle is what our essence is powering. There are three components I relate to when it comes to the vehicle, which should all look familiar to you at this point. They are:

1. The Physical Component - External Physical Body
2. The Systemic Component - Internal Systems of Body
3. The Mental Component - Our Operating System

Although each of these have unique characteristics individually, they all operate interdependently with one another. You cannot affect one without affecting the others. By now, you know I refer to these three components as the Trilogy of Vitality. Movement principles impact the external physical body—physical component. The vitality nutrition principles correlate to the internal systems of the body— systemic component. The mindset principles correlate to the operating system—the mental component. It is within these three components and the management of them where vitality becomes possible. One thing that has become abundantly clear working with thousands of individuals over the last twenty-plus years, is that one of these components has the ability, to most powerfully, trump the other two. That component is the mental component.

The mental component truly drives everything. I refer to the mental component as the operating system, since it dictates everything we do. While our essence powers the vehicle, the operating system drives the vehicle. The following two case studies illustrate how powerful the mental component is, whether it is driving us towards vitality or somewhere else.

CASE STUDY

"Thank You Jimmy D"

I remember looking over the health history of an individual who was referred to me for support with some aches and pains. He had a desire to get into better shape. This gentleman happened to be in his early eighties, was retired military, and ran a successful company that imported and exported cheeses around the world. However, he had quite a rap sheet when it came to his health history. The body diagram I use for clients to mark aches and pains was completely covered. I'm not sure there was a joint on this man's body that wasn't symptomatic.

He also added an additional page to indicate all the medications he was taking. My first surprise was when he walked into my clinic on his own and wasn't in a wheelchair. He didn't even use a cane! After completing his movement assessment, it was safe to say that the man's body had been through the ringer. I'm not sure you could have even called the things on the ends of his legs feet, they had been banged up so badly over the years. The number of biomechanical limitations this gentleman had and the amount of medication he was taking would have easily justified his being in a wheelchair or even bedridden. Well, not Jimmy D! He was the epitome of how a strong mental mindset can influence the body.

Every time Jimmy D came into the clinic, it was like a beam of light entered the space. He was always smiling and so happy and grateful to be there. His attitude and willingness to keep moving forward enjoying every moment was inspiring. As I got to know Jimmy D, I learned about his life and how it hadn't been an easy ride. He shared one story about the Korean War. He was a gunner. His plane took on enemy fire and started going down. In that moment, he believed he was going to die, and when his pilot somehow got them out of the tail spin and safely on the ground, nothing in his life was the same. After that event, he looked at life through a completely new lens and saw how every day was a gift and an opportunity to live his life to the fullest, pursuing what was most important and meaningful to him. He came from a very poor family and most of the time they all lived hand to mouth. After the war, he started a business that supported his siblings and extended family. He was able to provide them a life full of opportunities, education, and resources that no one in his family had ever before accessed.

The mental component was Jimmy D's big rock, and when I met him, he already had an incredible handle on it. I learned that my role was to simply augment and support his physical body as much as possible to complement what he was already doing.

Jimmy D is no longer with us today, but his memory clearly lives on. I am grateful to him for showing me the power of the mental component and the little talks that I had with him during those years still inspire me today. Thanks again, Jimmy D!

CASE STUDY

"Wait . . . what happened?"

Another case I will never forget that showed me the power of the mental component was a woman in her late fifties who was referred to me for some shoulder pain. She was someone who was relatively active, worked out consistently, and was still raising her teenage son and daughter. When I was evaluating her health history, there wasn't much there indicating serious biomechanical restrictions, besides the usual muscle soreness that many people have. One thing I noticed was that her neck, knee, and back were all areas where she indicated joint pain. This made me think the Power Regions might be her Big Rock and the place I would probably be starting. She had documented a typical day of eating which I looked at. I saw that she ate a very healthy diet, even by my standards. On top of all this, when she walked into my clinic she looked healthy and actually quite fit. I thought this was going to be a relatively easy case because shoulder pain, when biomechanically driven, is one of the easier cases to resolve for people.

As you are probably suspecting, it wasn't. When I meet someone the first time, I always spend the first 20–30 minutes really trying to understand the ins and outs of what a client is presenting. During this interaction, I ask a few key questions that address musculoskeletal pain.

1. How long have you had the symptom?
2. Do you remember anything happening that would have caused it?
3. Is there a specific position or motion that aggravates it?

After asking these questions, her report got a little more ambiguous regarding what was happening. She said she had the symptoms on and off for about a year, there wasn't any specific position or motion that aggravated her pain, and she couldn't recall any specific thing she did that would have caused it. I performed a simple range of motion assessment on her shoulder to see if there was a position that was limited or caused discomfort... nothing. When someone is experiencing non-specific pain that hurts randomly and is not tied to any position or motion, it is usually an indication that it may not be a mechanical problem, but rather something else may be driving the pain. I began digging deeper. I asked her about the marks I noticed she made on her neck, low back, and knees and asked her the same questions. Same answers—non-specific pain and no correlation to any position or motion. The only thing that was consistent was that all these symptoms started around the same time. So I probed a little more by asking her if anything significant happened in her life about a year ago. I was wondering if she had been in a car accident or something like that and forgot to tell me (wouldn't be the first time someone forgot something like that). She couldn't remember anything significant happening in her life a year ago but then added, very nonchalantly, "Well, I did find my mom dead in our pool about a year and a half ago." To which I said, "Wait . . . what did you say happened?" I thought I

might have misheard her, but I didn't. *DING! DING! DING!*
It looked like we found the BIG ROCK!

She asked me if I thought that this event may have had
something to do with all the non-specific pain and aches
she had all over her body. I absolutely did think there was
a correlation and wondered if she ever talked with someone
about the event and worked through the trauma of discovering
her mom dead in the pool. She had not because she stated
that there was no big emotional response. "I accepted what
happened, and moved on," she told me. This is a perfect
example of what happens when we suppress emotions and
never learn how to integrate them properly as we covered in
the previous chapter.

I didn't have the tools at that time to help her so I
encouraged her to talk with a therapist to help her integrate that
experience in a healthy way. I told her I'd be happy to do some
bodywork on her as a complement to working with a therapist
if she felt like it would be helpful, but that I didn't think her
symptoms were driven from biomechanical dysfunction.

This is one of many cases I have seen where the
suppression of emotions from a traumatic event or the
suppression of emotions as a coping mechanism over an
individual's lifetime, manifests as disease and dysfunction
in the body. Some of the more common ailments I found
to be correlated to unresolved suppressed emotions are non-
specific low back pain, shoulder and neck pain.

Needless to say, if the mental component is not aligned
with vitality, nothing else will be.

The Environment

The final player that we engage with each and every day is our
environment. This consists of the people, places, and things in

our life. Each one of these pieces is something we need to learn to leverage and align to help us fulfill our mission and purpose. We don't want to be dependent on our environment and we don't want to operate independently of our environment.

The sweet spot is to be interdependent with the environment and learn how to work with it—to be in coherence with it. As Dr. Stephen Covey said perfectly, *"Human life is interdependent! We can combine our talents and abilities and create something greater together."*[50] Being interdependent means having a solid foundation that we can stand on and leverage the capacities and talents of others and the environment to augment us on our journey.

The biggest resources that exist in our environment, in our three dimensional world, that we must learn to align with in order to fulfill our life's mission are:

1. Relationships
2. Money
3. Time
4. Things

Relationships

Relationships are big because they correlate directly with our biological need to belong and be accepted. Understanding how to properly integrate these needs as adults and evolve past the needs we had as children is the key to successful adult relationships. When we operate in the world as adults with a child's need to be accepted and loved, we create a lot of destruction and suffering for ourselves and others.

---

[50] Covey Stephen (2020)

Jim Rohn famously said that you are the average of the five people you spend the most time with.[51] This could not be better stated. The relationships you are involved with today are either supporting your fulfillment of your life's mission and purpose or they are inhibiting it. Doing an assessment on your current relationships and identifying where these relationships fall as far as your mission and purpose are concerned is essential to moving forward. This is an exercise we take individuals through in our *AIM Course*. Go to www. healthtovitality.com/AIM, for more details.

This doesn't always mean you must eliminate people from your life, although in some cases it may be a good idea. It usually is a combination of spending more time with people that support and align with your vision, less time with those that don't, and showing up in all of your relationships in ways that align with who and what you want to be.

This can be as simple as only engaging with a partner, friend, or family member when they are acting and behaving in alignment with the experience of the relationship you are looking to create. I have coached individuals who have partners who get angry, frustrated, and throw what I call adult temper tantrums. They can even become accusatory and demeaning in these circumstances. The strategy in these situations is to do your best not to engage. Not engaging means don't fight back and don't get into debates, arguments, and discussions when someone is behaving this way. Easier said than done at times, but if you can restrain yourself, take a deep breath and walk away, it offers the best option to allow the situation to cool off. Believe it or not, your partner wants to connect with you more than argue with you. The problem is that arguing has become the way of connecting

---

[51]   Rohn Jim in Groth Aimee (2012)

in many of these scenarios. Until you break the argument connection by no longer engaging, there will be no space to create a different type of connection. The other part of this strategy is to go out of your way to connect with them in alignment with the vision you have for the relationship when they are not angry or irritated. Show up with love, kindness, passion, and playfulness in those moments. This will eventually turn into a new place for positive connection to happen.

Time

As I alluded to earlier in the book, time is finite and we will never get back any day or moment we have already lived. My son Christian asked me a question recently. He said, "Dad, if I gave you $86,000 every day but whatever you don't spend, you lose, would you spend all of it?" I said, "I certainly would". To which he replied, "Well that's how many seconds we have each day, why don't we think about it the same way?"

Time is by far your most precious resource. It is essential to start believing your time is more valuable than money. Most people have this backwards. Time is a more valuable resource because it is a limited resource. You can always make more money; you can't make more time.

Managing your time is one of the most important skills to develop in order to create the most fulfilling and meaningful life possible. The absolute best way to manage time is to make your calendar and schedule into your best friend. I find that people have one of two types of relationships with their calendar. They either love it and live by it or dread the thought of having one. For those of you who cringed when I said your calendar and schedule need to be your best friend, I'd venture to guess it is because you associate calendars and schedules with restrictions and something that robs you of your freedom. I am going to invite you to start relating to your calendar a little differently. I suggest looking at your calendar as the tool that gives you your freedom. The way I relate to my calendar ensures that there is always time for me to do the things that are most important to me. The twelve-week chunk strategy is an excellent tool to help you manage your calendar, providing you with the assurance that you are able to do whatever things you value the most. In the *HABITS Course*, we take people through a time management system that ensures you have more than enough time to get the most important things done. For more information, go to www.vitalityprinciples.com/Habits.

Money

Although time is the most valuable resource, we all know money is a necessity. Whatever your mission and purpose is, money will most likely be a resource that you will need to leverage. Your relationship with money and the systems you have in place to manage money could be the difference between fulfilling your mission and purpose or not. This was a space I used to struggle with. I used to say, "I wish I could just do what I love doing and not have to worry about money." I also assumed people who had wealth were people who took advantage of others. I had a strong limiting belief that if your mission revolved around serving other people, it wasn't OK to earn too much money. Until I shifted that belief to understanding money is nothing more than a resource and that it was something I could leverage to serve and support more people, I struggled with money.

I am more financially stable today than I ever have been; it is a direct result of this shift in mindset. Looking at money as a resource to create the life and impact that was most important to me, rather than the ultimate goal, was the key shift.

Today when coaching people to create financial stability and build wealth over time, the first thing I ask them is how much money they want to make. For some strange reason, the standard response is about $10,000 a month or six figures a year. I find it fascinating that so many people felt this was the magic number. I'd follow up with, why $10,000? And the answer was usually that it seemed like it would be enough to pay the bills and have some left over. This is an example of a goal or target that is not specific enough, which makes achieving it very challenging. There is a principle called Parkinson's law that states, "work expands so as to fill the time available for its completion."[52]

I have found the same is true for money. If I have certain spending habits that leave me with no money left over at the end of the month, whether I have spent $5,000 or $20,000, I'm left with the same result. The other goal people will tell me is that they want to make "more money." This is another major trap because you named a destination that does not exist—no matter who you are, you can always make more money.

I was working with a client who desired to build her real estate portfolio to reach two million dollars. I took her through a process to create the strategies and action items that were most important for her to do to fulfill that outcome. Over the next six months, she accelerated herself to that number a lot faster than she anticipated. We got on a call together and she told me that she wanted to change her number to five million dollars. I asked her why she wanted to change it to five million and she answered, "Well, isn't more better?" This is an example of the "more" trap that

---

[52] Northcote Parkinson Cyril (1955)

never ends. We spent that session getting more clarity on what she actually wanted and what she was looking for the money to provide. She said she wanted financial security, meaning that her expenses were covered by her investments, and she could work if she wanted to, not because she needed to. We calculated the amount of money she needed annually to live the kind of lifestyle she was living and multiplied that by the amount of years she believed she would live. I then advised her to meet with a few financial planners to get some perspective and thoughts on the strategy she needed to create in order to fulfill that outcome. Turned out she was only about $500,000 dollars away from hitting the number she needed for financial security.

The key to creating a way to leverage money is to look at it as a resource, not the goal. The first thing I do with someone who comes to me for help with their financial goals, like the lady above, is to get them to focus on the lifestyle that is most important for them to know. Lifestyle includes everything from where you want to live, how big your house is, how you want to decorate your house, and what kind of car you want to drive all the way to the quality of food and your activities and hobbies.

I remember sitting down with Eve almost ten years ago and brainstorming everything we wanted to have in our lifestyle. At that time we named what we felt were outlandish things like getting regular massages, having a personal trainer, taking yearly family trips, creating certain opportunities for our two children, and eating nothing but the highest quality foods. I remember looking at the list and thinking we'd have to be millionaires to live this life. After doing the due diligence and calculating the cost of all of these things, it turned out it would cost us about $13,000 per month or a little more than $150,000 a year. That was a far cry from how I was relating to it. Just like it had for my client, all of a sudden it became something that was possible, and we actually weren't that far away from the reality of having enough money to live our desired lifestyle.

The power of this exercise was getting us to a place where we were not just focused on "making more money" or some ambiguous amount that we pulled out of thin air. It got us focused on what we really wanted, what was really important to us, the lifestyle that would be possible when we hit $13,000 a month—the exercise was inspiring and motivating.

A mentor once told me that your money lags twelve months behind your mindset, and I can attest to this being 100 percent accurate. The change in mindset I made around money over ten years ago has not only created the financial stability I know today, but for the first time in my life I am making consistent and steady progress toward building wealth.

Here is a very basic formula that you can use to get started on allocating your money to create financial stability and create wealth over time. There are many different ways to intricately allocate your finances depending on your situation and goals, but this breakdown is a good place to start if you have no system currently.

10% income long-term savings
This is money you put aside and forget it's there. It's money that goes into long-term investing—money you don't need for at least ten years that is earning a return for you year after year.

10% income short-term savings
This is for money that you may need in the short term, within six months to a year. This includes things like vacations, a new washer and dryer, or tires for your car.

It is highly recommended that you keep a minimum of six months of your lifestyle expenses in this account as a cushion.

80% income to lifestyle
This money is allocated to your lifestyle expenses which are things that you engage with on a monthly basis. This includes rent or mortgage, groceries, cars, insurance, hobbies, and so on.

Things

Oh, the things—so many things accumulate over the course of our lives and they all seem so important at the moment we acquire them. There is definitely nothing wrong with having things. The key is to use the things to augment and support you in creating your meaningful and purposeful life. Be mindful of when things become what gives us meaning and value. This is when we become enslaved to the things in our life hoping that more things will make us feel like we are enough. There are never enough things that we can accumulate that will make us feel like we are enough.

The best thing to do when looking to acquire something is to go through a few steps:

1. Do I have the money in my short-term savings account to buy this?
2. Is this something I need or want?
3. How does this contribute to moving me closer to my goals, mission, or purpose?

If the answer to step one is, "No, I don't have the money in my short-term savings account" then do everything in your power to do without the item. One thing that tends to fall into this category for people is eating out. It is one thing if you budget a certain amount of money toward dining out each month, it's another thing if you are spending money eating out and you have food in your fridge. Eve and I love trying new restaurants as part of our lifestyle. Therefore, we allocate a certain amount of money each month toward eating out. There are rare exceptions when you actually need to leverage credit cards to meet a need, but this should be the exception and a temporary situation as you build your short-term savings cushion.

If the answer to number one is yes, then ask the next question, is this something I need or want? Let's define a need. Need to me is something that directly impacts the lifestyle that I am currently living inside of the 80:20 model. Examples of needs are things that need to be replaced or repaired like appliances, cars, house, and so on. Other things in this category are really up to you and how you define what you need. For some people, their weekly massage is a need to maintain the vitality and energy necessary to fulfill their goals. I recommend taking some time and identifying your lifestyle needs *before* being faced with the question, is this thing a need? This will give a set of guidelines and an idea of how much your base lifestyle really costs and where you could trim some fat if necessary.

If the answer is, "it's just something I want," I recommend a few steps. First, sleep on it and see if you still want it in the morning. And two, make a rule that if you don't have at least a certain amount of money in your short-term savings (maybe that six months' worth of lifestyle expenses) then you will wait to purchase it.

The last question you want to ask is how this purchase or thing impacts your goals, mission, and purpose that you have named for yourself. Be honest with yourself. It is going to be one of two answers, it is moving you closer or moving you further away. This is one of the most important reasons to have your mission, purpose, and goals laid out and identified because they become your reference point to making decisions just like this. Having this reference point prevents you from making reactive decisions and deciding in a specific moment, "Oh, I didn't realize I needed that until right now."

CASE STUDY

"It's Never Too Late"

I was very fortunate to have two amazingly inspiring women come to me for some support with their bodies and eventually their minds. Both of these women were in their mid-eighties and still going after life in a big way. Their names were Marynance and Gloria. Both were active with consistent walking and even dancing at times. They also were very conscious about what they were eating. But like many individuals in their later years of life, they both struggled with the anxiety and fears of witnessing their bodies age a little bit more every year—not that this ever stopped them from showing up. They both came to the Vitality Center in Los Angeles for support with their bodies and engaged in bodywork, stretching, and some of the movement classes we offered.

Honestly, I underestimated both of them. When I asked them if they'd be interested in some of the mindset courses I was teaching, I didn't expect them to say yes. Boy, was I wrong. It looked like these two were already aware of their Big Rock and jumped on the opportunity to get their mindset aligned with all they were doing for their physical and systemic systems. They both pounced on the opportunity and dove in head first. I was amazed at how willing they were to go through the exercises and implement the steps - many of which were not exactly easy. Exercises and practices that required deep reflection on their past, and exploring and acknowledging ways of being, habits, and thoughts that didn't align with their goals.

Gloria had made her living doing commercial art. Her comment was "I just worked at it, to make my living." She struggled with some structural limitations in her spine. We calibrated and strengthened her mindset so she could continue being active with her movement, enjoy her painting, and learn more about different computer programs—which was something that very much intimidated her when she began. As a result of engaging with Gloria, I have two of her paintings hanging in my home. One of the paintings is of my son when he was about 2 years old and the other is a painting of my daughter around the same age. (Fig 39)

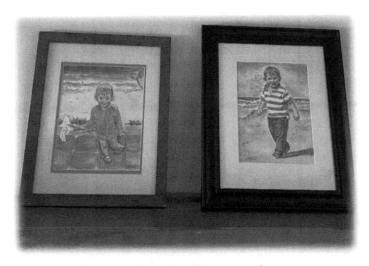

Fig 39: Paintings by Gloria Best of my son
Christian and daughter Emma.

One of Marynance's struggles was the idea that she was a witness to her life rather than the person in charge of it. She grew up in a generation where women didn't have the same opportunities and space available to live the life most meaningful and purposeful to them. Most of the time they were expected to "stay in their place" and fulfill the roles that were laid out for them. She said she felt as if a huge manhole cover called "I can't" was weighing down on her head all the time, yet she abounded in creativity and was always incredibly gifted with words. She had an insatiable curiosity for life and thirst for knowledge. Most of the time she kept her talents hidden, believing she had nothing to offer of commercial value. She only shared her gifts through her extensive volunteer work and never made any effort to share them through the marketplace due to a fear of failure, rejection, and ridicule, denying that she was an artist or a poet. As a result of leaning in and implementing some of the mindset principles from this chapter, Marynance, at the age of eighty-eight, compiled and published the first book of her poetry and is working on compiling several more. (Fig. 40) She has reclaimed her joy in painting, laughingly calls herself the Reluctant Poet, and is now in the process of compiling the second book of her poetry.

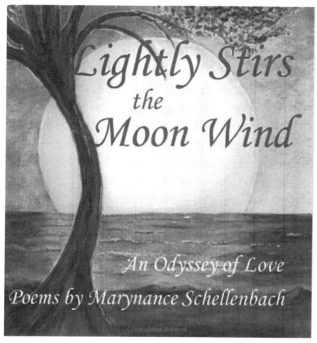

Fig 40: Marynance's first published book of poetry. And yes, the cover is one of her paintings

Gloria and Marynance will always live in my heart as inspiration for what is possible. They have proven to me that it is never too late to live the life we came here to live and are amazing examples of how to squeeze every last drop of life out of life.

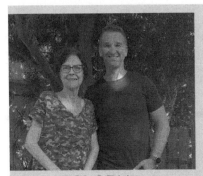

GLORIA

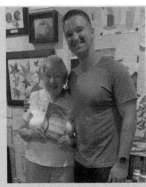

MARYNANCE

Current Day

Eve and I ended up selling our clinic in Southern California in 2017 to be closer to family living on the East Coast. Today, we live in beautiful Southern Florida with our two children Christian and Emma. I continue to work with individuals in my private practice from all over the world inside all aspects of The Trilogy of Vitality. I personally specialize in working with people in the movement and mindset components, while Eve has continued to dive into the systemic component. She has integrated other modalities to complement the nutritional component like homeopathy and energy work. She specializes in working with women struggling with hormonal imbalances.

To say our journey together has been adventurous would be an understatement. We just recently celebrated our twenty-year wedding anniversary in the Florida Keys. The laughter, joy, connection, and intimacy that we are experiencing twenty plus years into our relationship together has never been stronger.

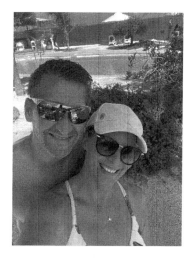

I am eternally grateful to have been blessed with the teachers, mentors, and role models in my life that have provided me with the resources to write and share "Health to Vitality" with you. My hope is that you have found some nuggets in this book that you can immediately start to apply, so you too can experience more Vitality in your life.

Want some individualized support and guidance implementing the content of this book?

If you are committed to empowering yourself with the Vitality Principles in this book and ready to create the life you are here and deserve to live, book a call using the link below and find out how you can get a customized plan and work directly with Matt and Eve.

HealthtoVitality.com/CommittedtoVitality

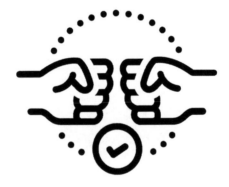

BONUSES!

MAKE SURE TO WATCH THE BOOK SUMMARY VIDEOS BY GOING TO:

WWW.HEALTHTOVITALITY.COM/VIDEOS

If you have made it this far, not only have you covered a ton of ground, but it is clear that you are committed to owning your journey and stepping into higher levels of vitality. I hope you feel inspired and that the life you deserve to live feels more attainable than ever before. Remember that it is *never* too late to implement these principles and I guarantee that if you implement just a few of the principles in this book, you will absolutely know and experience more vitality in your life. These videos will take your level of understanding to another level. They are absolutely free. Enjoy!

GET ACCESS TO ALL THE RESOURCES THAT I MENTIONED IN THE BOOK BY GOING TO:

WWW.HEALTHTOVITALITY.COM/RESOURCES

Resources include:

- Power Region Program Videos
- Vitality Big 6 Tracking Form
- Vitality Foundational Recipes
- Essence Meditation
- Purifying The Air You Breathe

You will also find information on the four courses that were mentioned in the book, AIM, ALIGN, HABITS, & RELATIONSHIPS as well as a form that you can use to make a request to get more information about a specific topic.

Love this book? Don't forget to leave a review!
Every review matters, and it matters a *lot!*
Head over to Amazon or wherever
you purchased this book
to leave an honest review for me.
I thank you endlessly.

Bibliography

Alliance News via Comtex. "Statins Market 2022 Expected to Witness the Highest Revenue Growth Over Forecast Period to 2030." MarketWatch. (July 12, 2022). https://www.marketwatch.com/press-release/statins-market-2022-expected-to-witness-the-highest-revenue-growth-over-forecast-period-to-2030-2022-07.

Amadeo Kimberly. "How Farm Subsidies Affect the U.S. Economy." The Balance. (April 18, 2022). https://www.thebalance.com/farm-subsidies-4173885.

Aristotle cited by Upton Joseph, Janeka Ivo, and Ferraro Nalton. "The whole is more than the sum of its parts: Aristotle, metaphysical." 2014 Jan; 25(1):59-63. doi: 10.1097/SCS.0000000000000369.

Benazzouz Ahlem, Amirouche Farid, Rieta José, and Guilal Rima. "Knee injuries classification using sEMG and goniometric features during gait." ResearchGate. (October 2019). https://www.researchgate.net/figure/Knee-flexion-extension-and-muscle-activity_fig1_341294412.

Brookes Megan. "Processed Foods in Pregnancy May Be Tied to Autism." WebMD. (June 26, 2019). https://www.webmd.com/brain/autism/news/20190627/processed-foods-in-pregnancy-may-be-tied-to-autism.

Burke Gregory, Sprafka Michael, Folsom Aaron, Hahn Lorraine, Luepker Russell, and Blackburn Henry. "Trends in Serum Cholesterol Levels from 1980 to 1987

— The Minnesota Heart Survey." N Engl J Med 1991; 324:941–946. doi: 10.1056/NEJM199104043241402.

Covey Stephen. The 7 Habits of Highly Effective People. Simon & Schuster, UK Ltd (2020).

Crum Alia and Lyddy Chris. "De-stressing Stress: The Power of Mindsets and the Art of Stressing Mindfully." The Handbook of Mindfulness. Wiley-Blackwell (June 2013). https://www0.gsb.columbia.edu/mygsb/faculty/research/pubfiles/6010/II%2043%20Crum%20Lyddy.pdf.

Dix Megan. "Everything You Should Know About Oxidative Stress." Healthline. (September 29, 2018). https://www.healthline.com/health/oxidative-stress.

Dweck Carol in Morehead James, "Stanford University's Carol Dweck on the Growth Mindset and Education." OneDublin.org. (June 19, 2012). Retrieved November 26, 2019. https://onedublin.org/2012/06/19/stanford-universitys-carol-dweck-on-the-growth-mindset-and-education/.

Felton C, Crook D, Davies M, and Oliver M. National Library of Medicine (PubMed.gov). Arterioscler Thromb Vasc Biol. 1997 Jul; 17(7):1337–45. doi: 10.1161/01.atv.17.7.1337.

Frankl Viktor. "Man's Search for Meaning." Beacon Press. (2006).

"Gladstone Rethinks Stress with Mindset Expert Alia Crum." Gladstone Institutes. (April 15, 2016). https://www.youtube.com/watch?v=4z9clzqhCN0&t=1946s.

Google – Dictionary Box. "Definition of Health" (2022). https://www.google.com/search?q=health+defined.

Grand View Research. "Market Analysis Report." (2018). https://www.grandviewresearch(2018).com/industry-analysis/personal-development-market.

HeartMath® Institute. "A Deeper View of Intuition." (August 26, 2019). https://www.heartmath.org/articles-of-the-heart/a-deeper-view-of-intuition/.

"How to make stress your friend." Talk by McGonigal Kelly. TED Talks. (September 4, 2013). https://www.youtube.com/watch?v=RcGyVTAoXEU.

Link Rachael. "Why Do Beans Give You Gas?" Healthline. (March 18, 2021). https://www.healthline.com/nutrition/why-do-beans-make-you-fart.

Maloiy, G, Heglund N, Prager N, Cavagna L, Taylor, CR (20 February 1986). "Energetic cost of carrying loads: have African women discovered an economic way?" Nature. 319.

Maslow Abraham. "A Theory of Human Motivation." *Psychological Review*. (1943).

Maté Gabor. Compassionate Inquiry Self-Study Online Course Compassionate Inquiry®. (January 2019). https://compassionateinquiry.com/short-course/.

Maté Gabor and Neufel Gordon. "Hold On To Your Kids: Why Parents Need to Matter More Than Peers." Ballantine Books. (August 15, 2006).

Maté Gabor. "What is Compassionate Inquiry®?" Compassionate Inquiry®. (May 23, 2017). https://compassionateinquiry.com/the-approach/.

McCloud Saul. "What is psychology?" (2019). Retrieved from https://www.simplypsychology.org/whatispsychology.html.

Kilby C and Sherman K. "Delineating the relationship between stress mindset and primary appraisals: preliminary findings." Europe PMC Springerplus, March 15, 2016, 5:336. doi: 10.1186/s40064-016-1937-7.

Nietzsche, Friedrich. "On the Genealogy of Morality." Translated by Clark Maudemarie and Swensen Alan. Hackett Publishing, 1998.

Northcote Parkinson Cyril. "Parkinson's Law." *The Economist*. London. (November 19, 1955).

NPR. "Vioxx: The Downfall of a Drug [Series]." (June 10, 2005–November 12, 2007). https://www.npr.org/series/5033105/vioxx-the-downfall-of-a-drug.

Ovid and the Censored Voice. "History of Roman Exile." (2022). https://web.colby.edu/ovid-censorship/exile/history-of-roman-exile/.

Oxford Languages. "Definition of Health." (2022). https://www.oed.com/view/Entry/85020.

Oxford Languages. "Definition of Catabolism." (2022). https://www.oed.com/view/Entry/28662.

Peat Ray. "Food-junk and some mystery ailments: Fatigue, Alzheimer's, Colitis, Immunodeficiency" (1995). http://raypeat.com/articles/nutrition/carrageenan.shtml.

Peat Ray. "Glycemia, starch, and sugar in context." (2009). http://raypeat.com/articles/articles/glycemia.shtml.

Peat Ray. "Suitable Fats, Unsuitable Fats: Issues in Nutrition." (2007). http://raypeat.com/articles/articles/unsuitablefats.shtml.

Peat Ray. "TSH, temperature, pulse rate, and other indicators in hypothyroidism." (2007). http://raypeat.com/articles/articles/hypothyroidism.shtml.

Raju Kale and Roshan Deshmukh. "Gluten-Free Products Market." Allied Market Research®. (April 2020). https://www.alliedmarketresearch.com/gluten-free-products-market#:~:text=The%20gluten%2Dfree%20products%20market,causes%20inflammation%20in%20small%20intestines.

Rohn Jim in Groth Aimee. "You're The Average Of The Five People You Spend The Most Time With." Insider. (July 24, 2012). https://www.businessinsider.com/jim-rohn-youre-the-average-of-the-five-people-you-spend-the-most-time-with-2012-7.

Schuker B, Wittes J, Santanello N, Weber S, McGoldrick D, Donato K, Levy A, Rifkind B. National Library of Medicine (PubMed.gov). Arch Intern Med. 1991 Apr; 151(4):666–73. https://pubmed.ncbi.nlm.nih. gov/2012446/.

Sinclair Marshall. "Why the Self-Help Industry Is Dominating the U.S." Medium. (February 25, 2019). https://medium. com/s/story/no-please-help-yourself-981058f3b7cf.

Sinek Simon. "How to discover your 'why' in difficult times." TED Talks. (2020). https://www.ted.com/talks/simon_ sinek_how_to_discover_your_why_in_difficult_times. Accessed 7/25/2020.

Takakol Ahmed and Ishai Amorina. "Relation between resting amygdalar activity and cardiovascular events: a longitudinal and cohort study." The Lancet. (2017).

The Free Dictionary. "Definition of Vitality" (2022). https:// www.thefreedictionary.com/vitality.

The University of Sydney. "Glycemic Index Research and GI News." (2022). https://glycemicindex.com/.

Tronick Edward (1975) in Goldman Jason. "The Research: The Still Face Experiment."

The Gottman Institute. (2022) https://www.gottman.com/ blog/research-still-face-experiment/.

Walden Michael "Human Skeleton: Planes Of Motion." TeachPE.com. (March 24, 2021). https://www.teachpe. com/anatomy-physiology/planes-of-movement.

Wikipedia. "Attachment Theory." (2022). https:// en.wikipedia.org/wiki/Attachment_theory.

Wikipedia. "Food Pyramid." (2022). https://en.wikipedia. org/wiki/Food_pyramid_(nutrition).

Wikipedia. "Locus of Control." (2022). https://en.wikipedia. org/wiki/Locus_of_control.